What Can I Do Now?

Health Care

Books in the
What Can I Do Now? Series

What Can I Do Now?

Health Care

Ferguson
An imprint of Infobase Publishing

What Can I Do Now? Health Care

Ferguson
An imprint of Infobase Publishing
132 West 31st Street
New York NY 10001

ISBN-10: 0-8160-6031-2
ISBN-13: 978-0-8160-6031-3

Library of Congress Cataloging-in-Publication Data

What can I do now? : Health care.
      p. cm.
  Includes index.
  ISBN 0-8160-6031-2 (hc : alk. paper)
  1. Medicine—Vocational guidance. I. J.G. Ferguson Publishing Company. II. Title: Health care.
  R690.W525 2007
  362.1023—dc22   2006030410

Ferguson books are available at special discounts when purchased in bulk quantities for businesses, associations, institutions, or sales promotions. Please call our Special Sales Department in New York at (212) 967-8800 or (800) 322-8755.

You can find Ferguson on the World Wide Web at http://www.fergpubco.com

Text design by Kerry Casey
Cover design by Takeshi Takahashi

Printed in the United States of America

VB Hermitage 10 9 8 7 6 5 4 3 2 1

This book is printed on acid-free paper.

All links and Web addresses were checked and verified to be correct at the time of publication. Because of the dynamic nature of the Web, some addresses and links may have changed since publication and may no longer be valid.

Contents

Introduction

If you are considering a career in health care—which is presumably the reason you're reading this book—you must realize that the better informed you are from the start, the better your chances of having a successful, satisfying career.

There is absolutely no reason to wait until you get out of high school to "get serious" about a career. That doesn't mean you have to make a firm, undying commitment right now. One of the biggest fears most people face at some point (sometimes more than once) is choosing the right career, and frankly, many people don't "choose" at all. They take a job because they need one, and all of a sudden 10 years have gone by and they wonder why they're stuck doing something they hate. Don't be one of those people! You have the opportunity right now—while you're still in high school and still relatively unencumbered with major adult responsibilities—to explore, to experience, to try out a work path—or several paths if you're one of those overachieving types. Wouldn't you really rather find out sooner than later that you're not cut out to be a physician after all, that you'd actually prefer to be a nurse practitioner? Or a medical writer? Or a genetic counselor?

There are many ways to explore the health care industry. This book gives you an idea of some of your options. Section 1, "What Do I Need to Know About Health Care?," provides an overview of the field—a little history, where it's at today, and promises of the future, as well as a breakdown of its structure (how it's organized) and a glimpse of some of its many career options.

Section 2, "Careers," section includes 10 chapters, each describing in detail a specific health care specialty: biomedical equipment technicians, diagnostic medical sonographers, genetic counselors, health advocates, health care managers, medical and science writers and editors, nurse assistants, nurses, physical therapists, and physicians. These chapters rely heavily on first-hand accounts from real people on the job. They'll tell you the skills you need, personal qualities you have to have, as well as the ups and downs of the jobs. You'll also find out about educational requirements—including specific high school and college classes—advancement possibilities, related jobs, salary ranges, and the employment outlook.

Section 3, "Do It Yourself," urges you to take charge and start your own programs and activities where none exist—school, community, or the nation.

The real meat of the book is in Section 4, "What Can I Do Right Now?" This is where you get busy and do something.

The chapter "Get Involved" describes volunteer and intern positions, summer camps and summer college study programs, and other opportunities.

While the best way to explore health care is to jump right in and start doing it (by volunteering at a hospital, doctor's office, etc.), there are plenty of other ways to get into the health care mind-set. "Surf the Web" offers you a short annotated list of health care Web sites where you can explore everything from job listings (start getting an idea of what employers are looking for now) to educational and certification requirements to on-the-job accounts.

"Read a Book" is an annotated bibliography of books (some new, some old) and periodicals. If you're even remotely considering a career in health care, reading a few books and checking out a few magazines is the easiest thing you can do. Don't stop with our list. Ask your librarian to point you to more health care-related materials.

"Ask for Money" is a sampling of health care scholarships. You need to be familiar with these because you're going to need money for school. You have to actively pursue scholarships; no one is going to come up to you in the hall one day and present you with a check because you're such a wonderful student. Applying for scholarships is work. It takes effort. And it must be done right and on time, often a year in advance of when you need the money.

"Look to the Pros" is the final chapter. It's a list of professional organizations that you can turn to for more information about accredited schools, education requirements, career descriptions, salary information, job listings, scholarships, and much more. Once you become a college student, you'll be able to join some of these. Time after time, professionals say that membership and active participation in a professional organization is one of the best ways to network (make valuable contacts) and gain recognition in your field.

High school can be a lot of fun. There are dances and football games; maybe you're in band or play a sport. Or maybe you hate school and are just biding your time until you graduate. Whoever you are, take a minute and try to imagine your life five years from now. Ten years from now. Where will you be? What will you be doing? Whether you realize it or not, how you choose to spend your time now—studying, playing, watching TV, working at a fast food restaurant, hanging out, whatever—will have an impact on your future. Look at how you're spending your time and ask yourself, "Where is this getting me?" If you can't come up with an answer, it's probably "nowhere." The choice is yours. It's up to you to choose your direction because, after all, it's your life. You can do something about it right now!

SECTION 1

What Do I Need to Know About Health Care?

The health care industry is the largest industry in the United States, employing 13.5 million people in 2004. Preventing, curing, and treating the diseases and injuries that affect the population is a major undertaking, requiring skill and training on every level. Read on for more information about this exciting, rewarding, and fast-growing occupational field.

GENERAL INFORMATION

The origins of medicine began with prehistoric people who believed that diseases were derived from supernatural powers. To destroy the evil spirits, they performed trephining, which involved cutting a hole in the victim's skull to release the spirit. Skulls have been found in which the trephine hole has healed, demonstrating that people did survive the ritual. The first doctors, known as medicine men, also used herbal concoctions, ritual dances, and incantations to heal their patients.

In about 3000 B.C., the ancient Egyptians developed a systematic method of treating illnesses, which introduced the notion of specialization within the field of medicine. The famous physician Imhotep was so respected that the Egyptians regarded him as the god of healing.

The Greek physician Hippocrates was the first person to declare that disease was caused by natural, not supernatural, phenomena. He introduced a method of conduct and ethics for the practice of medicine. To this day, each physician pledges the Hippocratic oath on the day of graduation from medical school.

Another Greek physician, Galen of Pergamum, studied in Rome during the second century A.D. He worked as physician to Emperor Marcus Aurelius and lectured to physicians on dissections and experimental physiology. He conducted anatomical studies of animals, particularly apes, because the dissection of humans was illegal. He is credited with the discoveries of blood transport by arteries, the pumping mechanism of the heart, and the function of the kidneys. His written work remained influential for hundreds of years, and during the 15th and 16th centuries, many physicians repeated his experiments to gain further insight into the mechanism of human anatomy.

Avicenna, from Persia, was another major contributor to the early development of Western medicine. His single largest contribution was the book *The Canon of Medicine,* which included the information of Greek and Arabic physicians that had been gathered from many generations, as well as some of his own findings. The book remained the most important publication for medicine through the 16th century and served as a major resource of information for Eastern and Western countries.

When dissection of human corpses was accepted in the 1500s, Andreas Vesalius was able to conduct his own examinations and correct many of the errors that Galen had made. Vesalius published *On the Structure of the Human Body* in 1543, which provided the base for future study of human anatomy.

William Harvey made an important contribution to medicine in the 17th century. Using the observations Hieronymus Fabricius had made on the valves in veins, Harvey conducted physical tests to prove that blood circulates through the body and through the veins and arteries. He wrote *On the Motion of the Heart and Blood in Animals* (1628).

It was the development of the microscope that moved medical study into the next plane of understanding. Zacharias Janssen, a Dutch eyeglass maker, discovered the benefits of combining magnifying lenses. He is credited with developing the first compound lens microscope around 1590.

Another Dutch scientist, Anton Van Leeuwenhoek, used microscopes to study the microscopic contents of water, blood, and other body fluids and tissues. He described bacteria from his observations, becoming the first person to recognize the presence of foreign bodies in human fluids.

Discoveries were made more rapidly once the concept of germ infection became recognized and accepted. The awareness of bacteria, fungi, and viruses led to concepts, taken for granted today, that proved to be a major boon to the medical profession. Washing hands before surgery, examinations, and deliveries of newborns led to a decrease in cases of infections and death. Joseph Lister developed the concept of an antiseptic environment that promoted sterilized equipment and surroundings in medical work.

Louis Pasteur successfully produced vaccinations that battled diseases. In the mid-1800s, Pasteur inoculated sheep against a common animal disease called

Lingo to Learn

ambulatory care Services for patients who are able to walk or move about.

HMO (health maintenance organization) A prepaid managed care plan that requires members to pay a fixed amount of money in exchange for most of their medical needs.

managed care A philosophy of health care that tries to keep medical costs down through education and preventive medicine.

outpatient Patient treated at the hospital but not admitted for extended care.

PPO (preferred provider organization) A health insurance plan that contracts with doctors, hospitals, and other providers to obtain discounts for medical care. The providers agree on a predetermined list of fees for all services. It is a form of managed care.

preventive care A type of medical care that stresses the prevention of disease by teaching patients better eating habits and other healthful lifestyle choices.

rehabilitation center A facility that uses therapy, education, and emotional support to help patients gain good health and lead useful lives.

residency A period of advanced medical training and education that is normally required after graduation from medical school.

stethoscope An instrument used for listening to sounds within the body, primarily in the heart and lungs.

anthrax. He went on to develop a vaccination against rabies, demonstrating that vaccinations were as successful in preventing disease in humans as they were in animals.

Another discovery that the modern world relies on every day is the development of anesthesia. Surgery had been performed without it for hundreds of years, but it was hazardous and extraordinarily painful. In 1846, a surgery by William Morton in Boston before a group of physicians proved to the medical world that the use of anesthesia freed the patient from surgical pain and allowed the physician to work more accurately, more thoroughly, and more extensively than ever before. Early anesthetics were nitrous oxide, ether, and chloroform.

Drugs were discovered that battled and killed some bacteria and infections. Alexander Fleming discovered penicillin in 1928. Howard Florey and Ernst Chain were able to isolate the penicillin compound in pure-enough quantities to use it to combat infections such as staph. That advance in 1938 led to mass production, which allowed the British and American armies to use it on wounded soldiers through World War II. The number of lives saved by penicillin is beyond calculation.

Immunologists and bacteriologists experimented with methods of inoculating soldiers against viral infections. Emil von Behring and Shibasaburo Kitasato developed tetanus antitoxin in 1890. The two also worked on diphtheria antitoxin, which, only after the vaccinations had a combination of toxins and antitoxins, would produce an immune response in humans.

During the 1930s, technology was developed that allowed immunologists to isolate and cultivate viruses for study and experimentation. As viruses were isolated, the proper vaccinations could be developed that would trigger immunization in humans. The most heralded of the vaccines was the one developed by Jonas Salk for poliomyelitis (polio). Albert Sabin developed an oral vaccine soon after, which also immunized against polio. Polio had infected hundreds of thousands of people in the United States between 1940 and 1959, and had killed 26,635 people, according to the National Center for Health Statistics. Initial use of the vaccination began in 1954. In 1960, thanks to the vaccination, only 3,190 Americans developed the disease.

Viruses still plague the population and therefore impact on the medical community. Acquired Immunodeficiency Syndrome (AIDS) is the most deadly virus to affect the population. By 2003, 524,060 people had died from AIDS in the United States, according to the Centers for Disease Control (CDC), and the disease had been diagnosed in 929,985 others. Severe acute respiratory syndrome (commonly known as SARS) is a viral respiratory illness that was first reported in Asia in 2003. Before the outbreak was contained, SARS spread to more than 24 countries in North America, South America, Europe, and Asia. According to the World Health Organization, 8,098 people worldwide contracted SARS during this outbreak and 774 of the group died. Beginning in late 2003, an outbreak of avian influenza, a virus that is carried by birds and occasionally transmitted to humans, also caused great concern for the medical community. Researchers are attempting to find a preventive vaccination and a cure for these deadly viruses.

The health care industry continues to develop at a rapid rate with the discoveries of new drugs, treatments, and cures. The medical community is using modern technologies, such as computers and virtual reality, to perform tests, compile data, diagnose illnesses, and train professionals. Many surgeries are no longer performed with a scalpel, but with lasers. Disease, illness, and injury are now being treated and cured so successfully that the general population is living much longer and the number of elderly is increasing.

Scientists are conducting promising research in the field of genetics. Knowledge about genes could help doctors identify people who have genetic predispositions to certain diseases and perhaps lead to a cure for such illnesses as Parkinson's disease and some types of cancer.

STRUCTURE OF THE INDUSTRY

Health care workers work in a variety of settings, including private offices, managed-care facilities, clinics, hospitals, research facilities, nursing homes, and private homes.

Private Offices

Physicians can operate a private practice, which may be an independent partnership or a group arrangement. Normally, office space is rented or purchased and diagnostic equipment also is purchased. The doctor will employ a staff, usually consisting of a receptionist and secretary, a nurse, and perhaps an X-ray technician or lab assistant. In group practice, three or more doctors will share the workspace and schedule hours that allow each some time off from emergency calls. In group practices, the doctors also share the cost of staffing, overhead, and insurance. Partnerships are the same arrangement as the group practice, with only two attending physicians. Other health care workers who have private or group practices include physical therapists, dentists, and nutritionists. Private practice is, however, becoming outmoded because of high costs of operation, and because more and more patients are becoming members of managed-care programs. Some health care professionals combine a private practice with part-time employment with a managed-care facility.

Managed-Care Facilities

The managed-care office, sponsored by health maintenance organizations (HMOs) and preferred provider organizations (PPOs), are the most popular health delivery systems today. The basic concept behind this structural arrangement is that patients pay a monthly fee instead of a fee-for-service arrangement. The treatments, within the limits of the provider package, are completely covered. So, for a regular monthly payment, basic health care is provided. PPOs may be arranged as a fee-for-service, which offer a reduced fee to patients signed up to use one (preferred) facility for their medical treatment. Managed-care facilities will offer the greatest number of employment opportunities for most health care professions in the next decade.

Clinics

Clinics function like a group practice. HMOs and PPOs sometimes use clinics for the provision of medical services, but other groups may also have clinics. The clinic is usually privately owned and is a profit-making organization. The number of employees may be quite large. The Mayo Clinic in Minnesota is one of the best-known clinics in the United States.

Clinics provide many of the services that a hospital provides as well as the general health care that a private practice physician provides. They may be equipped to do outpatient surgery (surgery that does not require an overnight stay), technical examinations and tests, and other complex procedures that the private office may not be able to do. Clinics may provide general care, with several different specialists on staff to handle the different aspects of health care, or they may specialize, with most of the physicians working in the same area of treatment.

Clinics may be affiliated with hospital facilities, universities, teaching centers, nonprofit organizations such as Planned Parenthood, or profit-making companies or partnerships. They are located all over the country.

Hospitals

Hospitals provide extended-stay health care for the ill or injured. They provide the broadest range of health care to the public. Hospitals may be run by private investors and owners, or they may be affiliated with an outside institution or organization. Universities, religious organizations, and the federal government sponsor hospitals. Community hospitals are normally nonprofit institutions. They provide service to the community at large, but they have become the most common treatment center for patients without medical insurance and those covered under Medicaid. Hospitals, like clinics, may cover general care or specialized care. Some hospitals have emergency wards where any emergency condition can be treated by emergency room physicians and surgeons. Other hospitals may specialize in maternity care, psychiatric treatment, drug dependency, or some other category of health concern. Long-term care is provided in nursing homes, psychiatric hospitals, hospices for the terminally ill, and general and special long-term facilities. In most large cities, there is at least one general care hospital. The cost of maintaining emergency room facilities, however, has reduced the number of hospitals that have sufficient staff to adequately handle emergency situations.

The number of hospitals in the United States peaked in the 1970s. There are fewer hospitals today because of hospital closings and consolidation of facilities. With the difficulty in maintaining a manageable budget, many hospitals have not been able to survive the rising cost of health care. For hospitals that serve uninsured patients, the lack of reimbursement has eroded the profitability of the institution. Federal, state, and locally sponsored hospitals have been the most likely to close. Rural hospitals may be the hardest hit by the rising cost of insurance and health care. The loss of a rural hospital may affect a larger area than the loss of an urban hospital, where the closest facility may be a few miles away. The rural patient may have to travel a hundred miles to find the nearest open hospital.

Research Facilities

Research is one of the most important areas of medical work. Biomedical research is funded by a variety of institutions, including manufacturers of pharmaceutical, electronic, chemical, and medical supply products; private health agencies, such as the American Cancer Society and the American Heart Association; endowments from philanthropic organizations; federal, state, and local governments; and hospitals, universities, and research organizations. Medical research offers employment opportunities to individuals with varying amounts of training, ranging from the researcher who possesses an advanced degree to the technicians and assistants who have high school or community college diplomas or a certificate from a laboratory technical school.

Many health care professionals perform research work in pathology laboratories or other types of laboratories. Health care professionals also work with architects, city planners, government officials, law enforcement officers, and highway engineers to solve such health-related problems as traffic safety, drug abuse, rodent control, and the design of appropriate and adequate community health facilities.

Other health care professionals research the problems concerned with the delivery of medical care services. They investigate such problems as why infant mortality and the incidence of tuberculosis is greater among some segments of the population than others. They search for ways to establish cooperative arrangements among various hospitals so that duplicate facilities for certain types of treatment do not exist where the area patient load requires only one facility. They work out the logistics of an efficient system of evening and weekend medical coverage for a community and design effective emergency teams trained in the latest methods of cardiopulmonary resuscitation.

Many research positions in health care are associated with teaching responsibilities, but opportunities for teaching exist at all levels in the health care professions. Opportunities exist in professional schools of medicine, nursing, dentistry, and veterinary medicine, and in the allied medical professions, including therapy occupations and medical technology.

Nursing Homes

The term "nursing home" usually makes people think of what are called skilled nursing facilities. These facilities provide 24-hour nursing care, meals, and living space to residents. However, other types of nursing or care facilities also exist. Intermediate-care facilities provide residents with meals and shelter and may also provide regular medical care, although not on a 24-hour basis. Residential care facilities, also called assisted living facilities, provide residents with meals and living space but offer only limited medical supervision and care. In addition to these three distinctions (skilled nursing, intermediate care, and residential care facilities), nursing homes can also be grouped into three categories based on their ownership. Not-for-profit nursing homes are run by voluntary organizations, such as fraternal or religious groups. Proprietary facilities are those run for profit by individuals, partnerships, or corporations. And government facilities are run, of course, by the government and include such places as veterans' homes and state-run nursing homes.

Home Care

Today, as patients spend less time in the hospital and as more medical procedures are done on an outpatient basis, the need for professional follow-up care in the home is essential. Recovery, rehabilitation, and care for illnesses and injuries are happening in the home. According to the Visiting Nurse Associations of America, home nurses care for nearly 4 million people every year.

CAREERS

It would take an entire volume to describe all of the careers available in the field of medicine and health. The following sections describe careers in the major segments of the health care industry.

Physicians

A *physician* may be a doctor of medicine (MD) or a doctor of osteopathic medicine (DO). Both may practice all accepted methods of treatment, including prescribing drugs and performing surgery, but the *osteopathic physician* places special emphasis on the body's musculoskeletal system with the underlying belief that good health requires proper alignment of bones, muscles, ligaments, and nerves. The principal medical practitioner is the doctor of medicine. There are more MD physicians than all other medical practitioners combined, including optometrists, osteopathic physicians, and podiatrists. The following paragraphs detail specialties in the medical field:

- *Allergists/immunologists* specialize in the treatment of allergic, asthmatic, and immunologic diseases. They treat patients with asthma, hay fever, food allergies, AIDS, rheumatoid arthritis, and other diseases.
- *Anesthesiologists* specialize in the planning, performance, and maintenance of a patient's anesthesia during surgical, obstetric, or other medical procedures. Using special equipment, monitors, and drugs, the anesthesiologist makes sure the patient feels no pain and remains uninjured during the procedure.
- *Cardiologists* practice in the subspecialty of internal medicine that concentrates on the diagnosis and treatment of heart disease. In most instances, cardiologists treat patients on a consultative basis to determine if the symptoms the patients are exhibiting are signs of heart disease.
- *Cosmetic surgeons* (also known as *plastic surgeons* or *esthetic surgeons*)

are medical doctors who specialize in surgeries to correct disfigurement and/or improve physical appearance. Though the terms cosmetic and plastic surgery are often used interchangeably, cosmetic surgery usually means procedures performed to reshape normal structures of the body to improve the patient's appearance. Plastic surgery generally refers to reconstructive surgeries performed on abnormal structures of the body caused by birth defects, developmental abnormalities, trauma, injury, infection, tumors, or disease.

- *Dermatologists* study, diagnose, and treat diseases and ailments of the skin, hair, mucous membranes, nails, and related tissues or structures. They may also perform cosmetic services, such as scar removal or hair transplants.

- An *ear, nose, and throat (ENT) specialist,* or *otolaryngologist,* provides comprehensive medical and surgical care for patients with diseases and disorders that involve or affect the ears, nose, throat, and related structures of the head and neck. Fifty percent of all physician office visits are for ear, nose, and throat illnesses. Many ENT specialists operate in private practices or work in large academic/university settings where they help train medical students and residents.

- *Gastroenterologists* specialize in the treatment of the digestive system and associated organs, like the liver and gall bladder.

- *General practitioners*, also known as *family practitioners*, see patients of all ages and both sexes, and will diagnose and treat those ailments that are not severe enough or unusual enough to require the services of a specialist. When special problems arise, however, the general practitioner will refer the patient to a specialist.

- *Geriatricians* have specialized knowledge regarding the prevention, diagnosis, treatment, and rehabilitation of disorders common to old age. The term "geriatrics" refers to the clinical aspects of aging and the comprehensive health care of older people. It is an area of medicine that focuses on health and disease in old age and is a growing medical specialty.

- *Holistic physicians* are licensed medical doctors who embrace the philosophy of treating the patient as a whole person. Their goal is to help the individual achieve maximum well-being for the mind, body, and spirit. Holistic medicine emphasizes a cooperative relationship between physician and patient and focuses on educating patients in taking responsibility for their lives and their health. Holistic physicians use many approaches to diagnosis and treatment, including alternative approaches such as acupuncture, meditation, nutritional counseling, and lifestyle changes.

- *Industrial physicians* or *occupational physicians* are employed by large industrial firms for two main reasons: to prevent illnesses that may be caused by certain kinds of work and to treat accidents or illnesses of employees. Although most industrial physicians may roughly be classified as general practitioners because of the wide variety of illnesses they must recognize and treat, their knowledge must also extend to public health techniques and to understanding such relatively new hazards as radiation and the toxic effects of various chemicals, including insecticides. A specialized type of industrial or occupational physician is the *flight surgeon.* Flight surgeons study the effects of high-altitude flying on the physical condition of flight personnel. They place members of the flight staff in special low-pressure and refrigeration chambers that simulate high-altitude conditions and study the reactions on their blood pressure, pulse and respiration rate, and body temperature.

- *Neurologists* diagnose and treat patients with diseases and disorders affecting such areas as the brain, spinal cord, peripheral nerves, muscles, and autonomic nervous system.
- *Obstetricians/gynecologists,* often abbreviated to *OBGYNs,* are physicians who are trained to provide medical and surgical care for disorders that affect the female reproductive system, to deliver babies, and to provide care for the unborn fetus and the newborn.
- *Oncologists* study, diagnose, and treat the tumors caused by cancer. When an individual is diagnosed with cancer, an oncologist takes charge of the patient's overall care and treatment

through all phases of the disease. There are three primary areas within clinical oncology: medical oncology, surgical oncology, and radiation oncology.
- *Ophthalmologists* specialize in the care of eyes and in the prevention and treatment of eye disease and injury. They test patients' vision and prescribe glasses or contact lenses. Most ophthalmologists also perform eye surgery, treating problems such as cataracts (which cloud vision) and other visual impairments. Because problems with vision may signal larger health problems, ophthalmologists may work with other physicians to help patients deal with diseases such as diabetes or multiple sclerosis.
- *Pathologists* analyze tissue specimens to identify abnormalities and diagnose diseases.
- *Pediatricians* provide health care to infants, children, and adolescents. Typically, a pediatrician meets a new patient soon after birth and takes care of that patient through his or her teenage years.
- *Podiatrists,* or *doctors of podiatric medicine,* diagnose and treat disorders and diseases of the foot and lower leg. The most common problems that they treat are bunions, calluses, corns, warts, ingrown toenails, heel spurs, arch problems, and ankle and foot injuries. Podiatrists also treat deformities and infections. A podiatrist may prescribe treatment by medical, surgical, and mechanical or physical means.

- *Psychiatrists* attend to patients' mental, emotional, and behavioral symptoms. They try to help people function better in their daily lives. Different kinds of psychiatrists use different treatment methods depending on their fields. They may explore a patient's beliefs and history. They may prescribe medicine, including tranquilizers, antipsychotics, and antidepressants. If they specialize in treating children, they may use play therapy.
- *Sports physicians* treat patients who have sustained injuries to their musculoskeletal systems during the play or practice of an individual or team sporting event. Sports physicians also do pre-participation tests and physical exams.
- *Surgeons* make diagnoses and provide preoperative, operative, and postoperative care in surgery affecting almost any part of the body. These doctors also work with trauma victims and the critically ill.
- *Urologists* specialize in the treatment of medical and surgical disorders of the adrenal gland and of the genitourinary system. They deal with the diseases of both the male and female urinary tract and of the male reproductive organs.
- Not all physicians treat patients. Some are in academic medicine and teach in medical schools or teaching hospitals. Some are engaged only in research.
- *Physician assistants* are not physicians, but practice medicine under the supervision of licensed doctors of medicine or osteopathy. They provide various health care services to patients. Much of the work they do was formerly limited to physicians.

Nursing

The largest group of workers in the health field are those in the nursing occupations: registered nurses, licensed practical nurses, nursing assistants, and psychiatric technicians. Depending on training and work setting, the nurse's job may include a wide range of duties related to caring for the sick or educating those who are well.

The two nursing career titles you may have heard of before you began researching the nursing field—registered nurse and licensed practical nurse—are the heart of the nursing field. Licensed practical nurses provide basic care to patients, often under the supervision of a registered nurse, and registered nurses can be found in areas from anesthetist nurses to emergency room nurses. You can aspire even further than registered nursing and become an advanced practice nurse. These nurses perform many of the duties normally restricted to doctors. Nursing assistants also make up a large part of the nursing personnel in most hospitals; this is a job that you can start during your summer vacations during high school, or right after graduation.

Psychiatric technicians work with mentally ill, emotionally disturbed, or developmentally disabled people. Their duties vary considerably depending on place of work, but may include helping patients with hygiene and housekeeping and recording patients' pulse, temperature, and respiration rates. Psychiatric technicians participate in treatment programs by having one-on-one sessions with patients, under a nurse's or counselor's direction.

Nursing assistants help registered nurses and licensed practical nurses with routine daily care of patients. Depending on where they are employed, nursing assistants may focus mainly on the physical needs of patients, such as helping them in and out of bed, admitting their paperwork, pushing their wheelchairs, and helping them walk. Some facilities also have nursing assistants who take and record blood pressure, pulse, temperature, and other vital signs.

Licensed practical nurses (*LPNs*), or *licensed vocational nurses*, give bedside care to sick, recovering, disabled, and injured patients in hospitals, clinics, nursing homes, and various other institutions. LPNs are required to have technical knowledge allowing them to perform tasks such as giving some medications, preparing and administering injections, and monitoring the patient's condition. They also record the patient's vital signs, assist the patient, and give general care in the form of wound dressing, compresses, and injections.

Registered nurses can work in a variety of settings. The workplace often defines the nature of the work for RNs. The following paragraphs list RNs in specific nursing careers.

Community health nurses, sometimes known as *public health nurses,* work in clinics, schools, and patients' homes to provide preventative health care, immunizations, health education, and nursing treatments prescribed by a physician.

Critical care nurses are specialized nurses who provide highly skilled direct patient care to critically ill patients needing intense medical treatment. Contrary to previously held beliefs that critical care nurses work only in intensive care units or cardiac care units of hospitals, today's critical care nurses work in the emergency departments, post-anesthesia recovery units, pediatric intensive care units, burn units, and neonatal intensive care units of medical facilities, as well as in other units that treat critically ill patients.

Dermatology nurses treat patients with diseases and ailments of the skin, hair, mucous membranes, nails, and related tissues or structures.

Emergency nurses provide highly skilled direct patient care to people who need emergency treatment for an illness or injury. Emergency nurses incorporate all the specialties of nursing. They care for infant, pediatric, adult, and elderly patients with a broad spectrum of medical needs.

Forensic nurses examine victims of crimes such as sexual assault, domestic abuse, child abuse, or elder abuse. They gather evidence and information for law enforcement officials. They may also gather evidence at crime scenes or in other settings.

Geriatric nurses provide direct patient care to elderly people in their homes, or in hospitals, nursing homes, and clinics. The term "geriatrics" refers to the clinical aspects of aging and the overall health care of the aging population. Since older people tend to have different reactions to illness and disease than younger people, treating them has become a specialty, and because the population is aging, the geriatric nurse is a promising nursing specialty.

Home health care nurses, also called *visiting nurses*, provide home-based health care under the direction of a physician. They care for persons who may be recovering from an accident, illness, surgery, cancer, or childbirth. They may work for a community organization, a private health care provider, or they may be independent nurses who work on a contract basis.

Hospice nurses care for people who are in the final stages of a terminal illness. Typically, a hospice patient has less than six months to live. Hospice nurses provide medical and emotional support to the patients and their families and friends. Hospice care usually takes place in the patient's home, but patients may also receive hospice care in a hospital room, nursing home, or a relative's home.

Hospital nurses follow the medical care instructions provided by the physician to care for the needs of the patients; this includes giving medications and treatments. Nurses also maintain patient records. RNs in this setting also instruct and supervise nursing staff in the bedside care of patients.

Neonatal nurses provide direct patient care to newborns in hospitals for the first month after birth. The babies they care for may be normal, they may be born prematurely, or they may be suffering from an illness or birth defect. Some of the babies require highly technical care such as surgery or the use of ventilators, incubators, or intravenous feedings.

Occupational health nurses work in businesses, government facilities, and factories to provide treatment for minor, on-the-job illnesses and injuries. Nurses also give physical examinations and provide educational sessions about workplace safety and health.

Office nurses assist doctors by preparing patients for examinations, performing laboratory testing, and overseeing administrative duties. These nurses may also work for dental surgeons, dentists, nurse practitioners, and nurse-midwives.

Oncological nurses specialize in the treatment and care of cancer patients. While many oncological nurses care directly for cancer patients, some may be involved in patient or community education, cancer prevention, or cancer research. They may work in specific areas of cancer nursing, such as pediatrics, cancer rehabilitation, chemotherapy, biotherapy, hospice, pain management, and others.

Psychiatric nurses focus on mental health. This includes the prevention of mental illness and the maintenance of good mental health, as well as the diagnosis and treatment of mental disorders. They care for pediatric, teen, adult, and elderly patients who may have a broad spectrum of mentally and emotionally related medical needs. In addition to providing individualized nursing care, psychiatric nurses serve as consultants, conduct research, and work in management and administrative positions in institutions and corporations.

School nurses give physical examinations to students; provide yearly visual, audio, and scoliosis screenings; and educate students, staff, and parents on child wellness issues.

Surgical nurses care for patients who are undergoing surgery. They include *floor nurses* (who work on surgical units) and *perioperative nurses.* There are several kinds of perioperative nurses. *Day surgery pre-op nurses* check patients in and get them ready for the day's surgery. *Scrub nurses* select and organize supplies and medical instruments that will be used during the surgery. The *circulating nurse* is a non-sterile member of the surgical team. Scrub and circulating nurses are also called *intra-op nurses. Post-anesthesia care unit nurses* take over from the intra-op nurses once the surgery is completed. They assess the patient for pain, breathing, bleeding, general vital signs, etc. They are also known as *post-op nurses* and *recovery room nurses.* Additionally, *RN first assistants* are a relatively new type of surgical nurse who work directly with surgeons in the operating room and in office settings seeing pre- and post-op patients. They may also check on pre- and post-op patients, but they are not floor nurses.

While RNs, LPNs, nursing assistants, and psychiatric technicians make up the greatest percentage of the nursing field, *advanced practice nurses* have higher training requirements and more responsibility. Nurse anesthetists, nurse-midwives, nurse practitioners, and clinical nurse specialists are examples of advanced

practice nurses. These advanced practice nurses have enough training and skill to do many of the tasks that are normally reserved for physicians.

- *Clinical nurse specialists* have higher training levels that are focused on a particular area, such as transplant nursing, critical care nursing, and cardiovascular nursing. Duties for these nurses vary depending on their specialty.
- *Nurse anesthetists* are among the highest paid in the nursing field. They administer anesthetics to patients prior to treatment or surgery.
- The *nurse-midwife* takes care of newborn babies and their mothers. The nurse-midwife spends much of the workday talking to and instructing new, or soon to be new, fathers and mothers.
- *Nurse practitioners* take on many of the responsibilities of a general physician. Nurse practitioners examine patients, take their histories, and diagnose and treat common medical illnesses and conditions.

Management

Health care managers organize and manage personnel, equipment, and auxiliary services. They hire and supervise personnel, handle budgets and fee schedules charged to patients, and establish billing procedures. In addition, they help plan space needs, purchase supplies and equipment, oversee building and equipment maintenance, and provide for mail, phones, laundry, and other services for patients and staff. In some health care institutions, many of these duties are delegated to assistants or to various department heads. These assistants may supervise operations in such clinical areas as surgery, nursing, dietary, or therapy and in such administrative areas as purchasing, finance, housekeeping, and maintenance.

Medical Technology

One of the most distinctive features of modern medicine is its increasing reliance on new and sophisticated pieces of medical machinery. New technology aids in making diagnoses, providing effective treatments, and taking over body functions when organs fail or patients undergo surgery. Because these new machines require special skills from the people who attend them, they provide opportunities for many new jobs. The following paragraphs detail careers in medical technology.

Biomedical equipment technicians handle the complex medical equipment and instruments found in hospitals, clinics, and research facilities. This equipment is used for medical therapy and diagnosis and includes heart-lung machines, artificial kidney machines, patient monitors, chemical analyzers, and other electrical, electronic, mechanical, or pneumatic devices.

Cardiovascular technologists assist physicians in diagnosing and treating heart and blood vessel ailments. Depending on their specialties, they operate electrocardiograph machines, perform Holter monitor and stress testing, and assist in cardiac catheterization procedures and ultrasound testing. These tasks help the physicians diagnose heart disease and monitor progress during treatment.

Diagnostic medical sonographers, sometimes known as *sonographers,* use advanced technology in the form of high-frequency sound waves similar to sonar to produce two-dimensional, gray-scale images of the internal body for analysis by radiologists and other physicians.

Dialysis technicians, also called *nephrology technicians* or *renal dialysis technicians*, set up and operate hemodialysis artificial kidney machines for patients with chronic renal failure (CRF). CRF is a condition where the kidneys cease to function normally. Many people, especially diabetics or people who suffer from undetected high blood pressure, develop this condition. These patients require hemodialysis to sustain life. In hemodialysis, the patient's blood is circulated through the dialysis machine, which filters out impurities, wastes, and excess fluids from the blood. The cleaned blood is then returned to the body. Dialysis technicians also maintain and repair this equipment as well as help educate the patient and family about dialysis.

Electroneurodiagnostic technologists, sometimes called *EEG technologists* or *END technologists*, operate electronic instruments called electroencephalographs. These instruments measure and record the brain's electrical activity. The information gathered is used by physicians (usually neurologists) to diagnose and determine the effects of certain diseases and injuries, including brain tumors, cerebral vascular strokes, Alzheimer's disease, epilepsy, some metabolic disorders, and brain injuries caused by accidents or infectious diseases.

Nuclear medicine technologists prepare and administer chemicals known as radiopharmaceuticals (radioactive drugs) used in the diagnosis and treatment of certain diseases. These drugs are administered to a patient and absorbed by specific locations in the patient's body, thus allowing technologists to use diagnostic equipment to image and analyze their concentration in certain tissues or organs. Technicians also perform laboratory tests on patients' blood and urine to determine certain body chemical levels.

Although *perfusionists*, formerly known as *cardiovascular perfusionists*, are not well known to the general public, they play a crucial role in the field of cardiovascular surgery by operating what is known as the heart-lung machine. The perfusionist is responsible for all aspects of the heart-lung machine whenever it becomes necessary to interrupt or replace the functioning of the heart by circulating blood outside of a patient's body.

Radiologic technologists operate equipment that creates images of a patient's body tissues, organs, and bones for the purpose of medical diagnoses and therapies. These images allow physicians to know the exact nature of a patient's injury or disease, such as the location of a broken bone or the confirmation of an ulcer.

Special procedures technologists are trained individuals who operate medical diagnostic imaging equipment such as computer tomography and magnetic res-

onance imaging scanners, and assist in imaging procedures such as angiography and cardiac catheterization.

Therapy/Rehabilitation

People working in therapy or rehabilitation help injured, disabled, or emotionally disturbed people regain their strength to the fullest extent possible. There are many different kinds of therapists, each with special knowledge and special skills. Some therapists, for instance, use dance, art, and music to help resolve patients' physical, emotional, and social problems. The following paragraphs detail careers in medical therapy and rehabilitation.

Art therapists treat and rehabilitate people with mental, physical, and emotional disabilities. They use the creative processes of art in their therapy sessions to determine the underlying causes of problems and to help patients achieve therapeutic goals. Therapists usually specialize in one particular type of therapeutic activity, such as painting, sculpture, or photography. The specific objectives of the therapeutic activities vary according to the needs of the patient and the setting of the therapy program.

Child life specialists work in health care settings to help infants, children, adolescents, and their families through illness or injury. One of the primary roles of the child life specialist is to ease the anxiety and stress that often accompany hospitalization, injury, or routine medical care.

Occupational therapists select and direct therapeutic activities designed to develop or restore maximum function to individuals with disabilities.

Average Hourly Earnings by Industry Segment, 2004

Establishment	Hourly Earnings
Hospitals	$20.31
Offices of dentists	$18.96
Outpatient care centers	$18.57
Offices of physicians	$18.41
Medical and diagnostic laboratories	$18.15
Offices of other health practitioners	$16.00
Home health care services	$14.41
Other ambulatory health care services	$14.32
Nursing and residential care facilities	$12.05

Source: U.S. Department of Labor

A *grief therapist* or *bereavement counselor* offers therapy for those who are mourning the death of a family member or a loved one. Therapists help survivors work through possible feelings of anger or guilt and help them recover from their loss. Counselors may be brought into communities or facilities to help individuals after a national disaster, act of violence, or an accident.

Horticultural therapists combine their love of plants and nature with their desire to help people improve their lives. They use gardening, plant care, and other nature activities as therapy tools for helping their clients to feel better by doing such things as focusing on a project, improving social skills, and being physically active. In addition to these benefits, clients experience emotional benefits, such as feeling secure, responsible, and needed.

Hypnosis is a sleep-like state brought on by another person's suggestions. It may be suggested to people under hypnosis that they relax, change their way of thinking, or even move under direction. *Hypnotherapists* help people use the power of their mind to increase motivation, change behavior, and promote healing.

Music therapists treat and rehabilitate people with mental, physical, and emotional disabilities. They use the creative process of music in their therapy sessions to determine the underlying causes of problems and to help patients achieve therapeutic goals. The specific objectives of the therapeutic activities vary according to the needs of the patient and the setting of the therapy program.

Occupational therapy assistants (OTAs) work under the direct supervision of an occupational therapist to aid in helping people with mental, physical, developmental, or emotional limitations learn a variety of activities to improve basic motor functions and reasoning abilities. Their duties include helping to plan, implement, and evaluate rehabilitation programs designed to regain patients' self-sufficiency and to restore their physical and mental functions. *Occupational therapy aides* help OTAs and occupational therapists by doing such things as clerical work, preparing therapy equipment for a client's use, and keeping track of supplies.

Orthotic technicians and *prosthetic technicians* make, fit, repair, and maintain orthotic and prosthetic devices according to specifications and under the guidance of orthotists and prosthetists. Orthotic devices, sometimes also referred to as orthopedic appliances, are braces used to support weak or ineffective joints or muscles or to correct physical defects, such as spinal deformities. Prosthetic devices are artificial limbs and plastic cosmetic devices. These devices are designed and fitted to the patient by prosthetists or orthotists.

Orthotists design and make braces, shoe inserts, and other corrective devices to support the spine or limbs weakened by illness or injury. *Prosthetists* design, make, and fit artificial limbs for persons missing an arm, leg, or other body part as a result of injury or illness.

Pedorthists design, manufacture, fit, and modify shoes and other devices aimed at lessening pain or correcting foot problems. Pedorthists design and fit special therapeutic footwear for a patient as prescribed by a physician. This process involves making clay impressions of the patient's feet, modifying the mold to make special footwear, choosing the correct materials, and, finally, creating the custom footwear.

Physical therapists, formerly called *physiotherapists,* are health care specialists who restore mobility, alleviate pain and suffering, and work to prevent permanent disability for their patients. They test and measure the functions of the musculoskeletal, neurological, pulmonary, and cardiovascular systems and treat problems in these systems caused by illness, injury, or birth defect. Physical therapists provide preventive, restorative, and rehabilitative treatment for their patients.

Physical therapy assistants help to restore physical function in people with injury, birth defects, or disease. They assist physical therapists with a variety of techniques, such as exercise, massage, heat, and water therapy.

Psychologists teach, counsel, conduct research, or administer programs to understand people and help people understand themselves. Psychologists examine individual and group behavior through testing, experimenting, and studying personal histories. Psychologists normally hold doctorates in psychology. Unlike psychiatrists, they are not medical doctors and cannot prescribe medication.

Recreational therapists plan, organize, direct, and monitor medically approved recreation programs for patients in hospitals, clinics, and various community settings. These therapists use recreational activities to assist patients with mental, physical, or emotional disabilities to achieve the maximum possible functional independence.

Rehabilitation counselors provide counseling and guidance services to people with disabilities to help them resolve life problems and to train for and locate work that is suitable to their physical and mental abilities, interests, and aptitudes.

Respiratory therapists, also known as *respiratory care practitioners*, evaluate, treat, and care for patients with deficiencies or abnormalities of the cardiopulmonary (heart/lung) system, either providing temporary relief from chronic ailments or administering emergency care where life is threatened. They are involved with the supervision of other respiratory care workers in their area of treatment. Respiratory technicians have many of the same responsibilities as therapists; however, technicians do not supervise other respiratory care workers.

Speech-language pathologists and *audiologists* help people who have speech and hearing defects. They identify the problem, and then use tests to further evaluate it. Speech-language pathologists try to improve the speech and language skills of clients with communications disorders. Audiologists perform tests to measure the hearing ability of clients, who may range in age from the very young to the very old. Since it is not uncommon for clients to require assistance in speech and hearing, pathologists and audiologists may frequently work together to help clients. Some professionals decide to combine these jobs into one, working as *speech-language pathologists/audiologists*.

Other Health Care Careers

Biomedical engineers are highly trained scientists who use engineering and life science principles to research biological aspects of animal and human life. They develop new theories, and they modify, test, and prove existing theories on life systems. They design health care instruments and devices or apply engineering principles to the study of human systems.

Dietetic technicians work in hospitals, nursing homes, public health nutritional programs, food companies, and other institutional settings that require food-service management and nutritional-care services. They usually work under the direction of a dietitian or nutritionist, as members of a team.

Emergency medical technicians, often called *EMTs*, respond to medical emergencies to provide immediate treatment for ill or injured persons both on the scene and during transport to a medical facility. They function as part of an emergency medical team, and the range of medical services they perform varies according to their level of training and certification.

Registered dietitians (RDs) are professionals who have met certain educational requirements and passed a national certification exam. For the purposes of this article, the terms "dietitian" and "registered dietitian" will be used interchangeably. RDs provide people with foods and dietary advice that will improve or maintain their health. They may be self-employed or work for institutions, such as hospitals, schools, restaurants, and nursing homes—any place where food is served or nutritional counseling is required. *Hospital dietitians,* for example, may ensure that the food served in the cafeteria is nourishing or create special diets for patients with particular nutritional problems and needs.

Health advocates, also known as *patient representatives* and *patient advocates,* work with and on behalf of patients to resolve issues ranging from getting insurance coverage to dealing with complaints about the medical staff to explaining a doctor's treatment plan.

Health care educators are needed to teach patient care, research techniques, surgical techniques, equipment operation and repair, and counseling/therapy techniques to health care students in classroom and clinical settings.

Histologic technicians perform basic laboratory procedures to prepare tissue specimens for microscopic examination. They process specimens to prevent deterioration and cut them using special laboratory equipment. They stain specimens with special dyes and mount the tissues on slides. Histologic technicians work closely with pathologists and other medical personnel to detect disease and illness.

Home health care aides, also known as *homemaker-home health aides* or *home attendants,* serve elderly and infirm persons by visiting them in their homes and caring for them. Working under the supervision of nurses or social workers, they perform various household chores

that clients are unable to perform for themselves as well as attend to patients' personal needs. Although they work primarily with the elderly, home health care aides also attend to clients with disabilities or those needing help with small children.

Hospice workers provide support for terminally ill patients in the final stages of their illness. Hospice care is a benefit under Medicare Hospital Insurance and eligible persons can receive medical and support services for their terminal illnesses. Care is primarily provided in the patients' homes, but may also be provided in nursing homes and hospitals, with the intent to make patients as comfortable and pain-free as medically possible during the final days of their lives. A team of specially trained professionals and volunteers provides hospice care.

Medical and science writers translate technical medical and scientific information so it can be disseminated to the general public and professionals in the field. Science and medical writers research, interpret, write, and edit scientific and medical information.

Medical assistants help physicians in offices, hospitals, and clinics. They keep medical records, help examine and treat patients, and perform routine office duties to allow physicians to spend their time working directly with patients. Medical assistants are vitally important to the smooth and efficient operation of medical offices.

Medical ethicists are consultants, teachers, researchers, and policy makers in the field of medical ethics, the branch of philosophy that addresses the moral issues involved in medical practice and research.

Medical laboratory technicians perform routine tests in medical laboratories. These tests help physicians and other professional medical personnel diagnose and treat disease. Technicians prepare samples of body tissue; perform laboratory tests such as urinalysis and blood counts; and make chemical and biological analyses of cells, tissue, blood, or other body specimens. They usually work under the supervision of a medical technologist or a laboratory director.

In any hospital, clinic, or other health care facility, permanent records are created and maintained for all the patients treated by the staff. Each patient's medical record describes in detail his or her condition over time. Entries include illness and injuries, operations, treatments, outpatient visits, and the progress of hospital stays. *Medical record technicians* compile, code, and maintain these records. They also tabulate and analyze data from groups of records in order to assemble reports. They review records for completeness and accuracy; assign codes to the diseases, operations, diagnoses, and treatments according to detailed standardized classification systems; and post the codes on the medical record. They transcribe medical reports; maintain indices of patients, diseases, operations, and other categories of information; compile patient census data; and file records. In addition, they may direct the day-to-day operations of the medical records department.

Medical technologists, also called *clinical laboratory technologists,* are health professionals whose jobs include many health care roles. They perform laboratory tests essential to the detection, diagnosis, and treatment of disease. They work under the direction of laboratory managers and pathologists.

Medical transcriptionists listen to tapes and transcribe, or type, reports of what the doctor said. The reports are then included in patients' charts. Medical transcriptionists work in a variety of health care settings, including hospitals, clinics, and doctors' offices, as well as for transcription companies or out of their own homes. Medical transcriptionists are also called *medical transcribers, medical stenographers,* or *medical language specialists.*

Nursing home administrators are responsible for the management of nursing homes. Their duties are wide ranging, covering everything from keeping track of financial accounts to making sure the facility is up to code to greeting residents at social events. In addition, administrators supervise managers throughout the residence.

Nursing home managers head different departments of a facility, such as housekeeping, dietary, human resources, and they report any problems or needs to the nursing home administrator, who then addresses the situation.

Nutritionists usually work in private practice and are concerned with the biochemical aspects of nutrition.

Surgical technologists, also called *surgical technicians* or *operating room technicians,* are members of the surgical team who work in the operating room with surgeons, nurses, anesthesiologists, and other personnel before, during, and after surgery. They perform functions that ensure a safe and sterile environment.

Transplant coordinators are involved in practically every aspect of organ procurement (getting the organ from the donor) and transplantation. There are two types of transplant coordinators: *procurement coordinators* and *clinical coordinators.* Procurement coordinators help the families of organ donors deal with the death of a loved one as well as inform them of the organ donation process. Clinical coordinators educate recipients about how to prepare for an organ transplant and how to care for themselves after the transplant.

Employment Opportunities

Opportunities in health care are available in hospitals, managed-care facilities, nursing homes and long-term health care facilities, doctors' offices, community health clinics, home health care, schools, health maintenance organizations, colleges and universities, prisons and correctional facilities, disaster relief organizations, and local, state, and federal governments.

Industry Outlook

According to U.S. government projections, employment in the health services industry is projected to increase 27 percent through 2014, adding about 3.6 million new jobs over the 2002-2012 period. Projected rates of employment growth for the various segments of this industry range

Employment in the Health Care Industry

Establishment	Employment (by percentage)
Hospitals, public and private	41.3
Nursing and residential care facilities	21.3
Offices of physicians	15.5
Home health care services	5.8
Offices of dentists	5.7
Offices of other health practitioners	4.0
Outpatient care centers	3.4
Other ambulatory health care services	1.5
Medical and diagnostic laboratories	1.4

Source: U.S. Department of Labor

from 13.1 percent in hospitals, the largest and slowest growing industry segment, to 69.5 percent in the much smaller, but fastest growing home health care services segment. The U.S. Department of Labor also says that 13 of the 20 occupations projected to grow the fastest are concentrated in the health services industry.

Employment for physicians and surgeons is expected to grow faster than the average. More doctors will be needed because the population is both growing and aging. Also, many new technological improvements require the expertise of greater numbers of medical specialists. The need for primary care providers, however, will be far greater than the need for medical specialists. Job prospects will be best in internal medicine, family practice, geriatrics, and preventive medicine.

Since managed-care programs are growing because of their cost efficiency, employment opportunities in hospitals are expected to decline, especially in administrative and support jobs. Some observers expect that consolidations and closings will reduce the number of community hospitals by as much as 10 percent. Remaining hospitals are likely to cut costs, reduce staff, curb the use of advanced technologies, encourage outpatient care, and reduce paperwork. In the next decade, most health care workers will be employed in some kind of corporate, group, or network environment.

One of the fastest growing job categories in the industry is home health care. Home health care workers include nurses, physical therapists, and consultants, as well as lower-paid workers who cook, clean, bathe, and dress homebound patients, such as the elderly and people with disabilities.

Opportunities are excellent for nurse practitioners and physician assistants, too. They will begin to assume many of the functions of primary care physicians in the next few years, including taking patient histories and making preliminary diagnoses.

The employment outlook for all kinds of nurses is very favorable. Many hospitals don't have enough nurses; the demand is bigger than the supply. Also, as health care services expand, even more nurses will be needed.

The employment outlook for physical therapists is also excellent. Occupational and physical therapy are expected to remain among the top growth careers in the United States. Other health care jobs with a promising outlook include dental assistants and hygienists, home health care aides, medical assistants, personal and home care aides, diagnostic medical sonographers, and medical scientists.

SECTION 2

Careers

Biomedical Equipment Technicians

SUMMARY

Definition
Biomedical equipment technicians install, maintain, repair, and calibrate biomedical equipment used in hospitals, clinics, and other medical or laboratory facilities.

Alternative Job Titles
Biomedical electronics technicians
Biomedical engineering technicians
Biomedical engineering technologists
Biomedical engineering technology specialists
Biomedical instrumentation technicians
Clinical engineering technicians
Field service engineers

Salary Range
$22,630 to $51,289 to $60,050+

Educational Requirements
Associate degree

Certification or Licensing
Voluntary

Outlook
About as fast as the average

High School Subjects
Chemistry
Computer science
Mathematics
Physics
Shop (trade/vo-tech education)

Personal Interests
Building things
Computers
Figuring out how things work
Fixing things
Science

Responding to a request for assistance, the biomedical equipment technician walks into the operating room to find a roomful of medical professionals staring in her direction. She's directed to the faulty equipment—an aortic balloon pump designed to assist the heart if it is not functioning correctly. The technician can't very well take the machine apart in the operating room, but she has diagnosed the problem. She exits the operating room, runs down two floors, grabs a new set of cables, and rushes back up. She plugs one end of the new cables into the machine, and it starts pumping as it should. The technician breathes a sigh of relief and leaves the operating room as the surgical team hurriedly resumes the operation. She heads back down to the equipment shop. Saving lives is all in a day's work for a biomedical equipment technician.

WHAT DOES A BIOMEDICAL EQUIPMENT TECHNICIAN DO?

Biomedical equipment technicians are an important link between technology and medicine. They repair, calibrate, maintain, and operate biomedical equipment, working under the supervision of researchers, biomedical engineers, physicians, surgeons, and other professional health care providers.

Biomedical equipment technicians may work with thousands of different kinds of equipment. Some of the most frequently encountered are the following: patient monitors; heart-lung machines; kidney machines; blood-gas analyzers; spectrophotometers; X-ray units; radiation monitors; defibrillators; anesthesia apparatus; pacemakers; blood pressure transducers; spirometers; sterilizers; diathermy equipment; telemetry systems; ultrasound machines; and imaging technology, such as the CT (computed tomography) scan machine, PETT (positive emission transaxial tomography) scanner, and MRI (magnetic resonance imaging) machines.

Repairing faulty instruments is one of the chief functions of biomedical equipment technicians. They investigate equipment problems, determine the extent of malfunctions, make repairs on instruments that have had minor breakdowns, and expedite the repair of instruments with major breakdowns, for instance, by writing an analysis of the problem for the factory. In doing this work, technicians rely on manufacturers' diagrams, maintenance manuals, and standard and specialized test instruments, such as oscilloscopes and pressure gauges.

Installing equipment is another important function of biomedical equipment technicians. They inspect and test new equipment to make sure it complies with performance and safety standards as described in the manufacturer's manuals and diagrams, and as noted on the purchase order. Technicians may also check on proper installation of the equipment, or, in some cases, install it themselves. To ensure safe operations, technicians need a thorough knowledge of the regulations related to the proper grounding of equipment, and they need to actively carry out all steps and procedures to ensure safety.

Maintenance is the third major area of responsibility for biomedical equipment technicians. In doing this work, technicians try to catch problems before they become more serious. To this end, they take apart and reassemble devices, test circuits, clean and oil moving parts, and replace worn parts. They also keep complete records of all machine repairs, maintenance checks, and expenses.

In all three of these functions, a large part of technicians' work consists of consulting with nurses, physicians, administrators, engineers, and other related professionals; for example, they may be called upon to assist hospital administrators as they make decisions about the repair, replacement, or purchase of new equipment. They consult with medical and research staffs to determine that equipment is functioning safely and properly. They also consult with medical and engineering staffs when called upon to modify or develop equipment. In all of these activities, they use their knowledge of electronics, medical terminology, human anatomy and physiology, chemistry, and physics.

In addition, biomedical equipment technicians are involved in a range of other related duties. Some biomedical equipment technicians maintain inventories of all instruments in the hospital, making detailed notes about their condition, location, and operators. They reorder parts and components, assist in providing people with emergency instruments, restore unsafe or defective instruments to working order, and check for safety regulation compliance.

Other biomedical equipment technicians help physicians, surgeons, nurses, and researchers conduct procedures and experiments. In addition, they must be able to explain to staff members how to operate these machines, the conditions under which certain apparatus may or may not be used, how to solve small operating problems, and how to monitor and maintain equipment.

In many hospitals, technicians are assigned to a particular service, such as pediatrics, surgery, or renal medicine. These technicians become specialists in certain types of equipment. Unlike electrocardiograph technicians or dialysis technicians, however, who specialize in one kind of equipment, most biomedical equipment technicians must be thoroughly familiar with a large variety of instruments. They might be called upon to prepare an artificial kidney or to work with a blood-gas analyzer. Biomedical equipment technicians also maintain pulmonary function machines. These machines are used in clinics for ambulatory patients, hospital laboratories, departments of medicine for diagnosis

---

Lingo to Learn

biomechanics Explores the response of living matter to physical forces, such as how the knee of a jogger responds to repeated impact on the pavement.

calibrate To adjust or set a device so that it records and measures accurately.

defibrillator An electronic device that creates an electric shock designed to restore the rhythm of a fibrillating heart.

fibrillation Irregular, rapid contractions of the heart muscles that cause the heartbeat and pulse to fall out of synchronism.

heart-lung machine A machine used to divert blood from the heart during heart surgery and to keep it oxygenated and in circulation.

metabolic imaging Noninvasive methods of seeing inside the body, such as positron emission tomography (PET), magnetic resonance imaging (MRI), X-ray computed tomography (CT or CAT scan), and ultrasound.

pulmonary function machine A machine that examines and measures a patient's breathing efficiency and analyzes the gases throughout the lungs.

---

and treatment, and rehabilitation of cardiopulmonary patients.

While most biomedical equipment technicians are trained in electronics technology, there is also a need for technicians trained in plastics to work on the development of artificial organs and for people trained in glassblowing to help make the precision parts for specialized equipment.

Many biomedical equipment technicians work for medical equipment manufacturers. These technicians, sometimes known as *field service engineers,* perform repairs and preventive maintenance for specific lines of equipment manufactured by their employer.

WHAT IS IT LIKE TO BE A BIOMEDICAL EQUIPMENT TECHNICIAN?

Dennis McMahon became a biomedical technician, like many of his colleagues in the '70s and '80s, through what he calls the "back door." "I was always interested in science and radio-electronics," he recalls, "and learned a great deal of electronics by self-study. As soon as I finished my degree in chemistry in 1968, I studied for and obtained an amateur radio operator's license and pursued that as a hobby. In the early 1970s, I was an anesthesia technician in the operating room of a major teaching hospital, which involves the application of a lot of technology in the surgical setting. After taking classes in basic electronics and changing employers, I wrote my CBET exam in March of 1980, and eventually assumed the role of biomed tech in the operating room. In a sense, my hobby became my job."

In addition to his duties as a biomedical equipment technician at Virginia Mason Medical Center in Seattle, Washington, Dennis teaches biomedical technology at North Seattle Community College. "In 2001, the instructor position for their biomedical technology classes became available," he says, "and I began co-instructing classes in the fall with another biomed from the local area. Our program features classes and labs in the fall and winter quarters, and the students then take an internship at local hospitals during the spring."

Unlike technicians who have more general duties, Dennis works in Perioperative Services, which includes surgery, anesthesiology, and the recovery rooms. "The first 90 minutes of my 'typical day,'" he says, "tend to have a series of calls to troubleshoot apparent equipment problems in the many surgery rooms, deal with set-up issues, or prepare specific equipment for procedures scheduled for later in the day. The balance of the day is a mixture of pursuing my assigned preventative maintenance procedures for the month, and dealing with random interruptions for troubleshooting and repairs. This can be a physical job. There is a lot of running up and down stairwells to get to the rooms where there are issues, and some days seem to involve a lot of lifting and bending. And any biomed work involves exposure to occupational hazards that are unique to health care: HIV, hepatitis B, resistant strains of staph, radiation, radioisotopes, and lasers."

Dennis says that he spends about half of his time performing scheduled preventative maintenance procedures and about a third of his time repairing equipment. "Documentation of all these activities is important for credentialing and legal purposes," he explains, "so paperwork accounts for at least another 10 percent of an average day."

Myron Hartman is an instructor and the program coordinator for Pennsylvania

To Be a Successful Biomedical Equipment Technician, You Should . . .

- be technically adept
- have good problem-solving skills
- be attentive to detail
- be a good communicator
- have the ability to work as a member of a team

State University's Biomedical Engineering Technology program, one of only two programs of its kind in the nation to be accredited by the Technology Accreditation Commission for the Accreditation Board for Engineering and Technology. "After working in the field for more than 22 years as a biomedical equipment technician, supervisor, manager, director, administrator, and part-time teacher," he says, "I decided to enter the teaching profession. I am currently in my fifth year of teaching biomedical engineering technology for Penn State University at the New Kensington campus."

DO I HAVE I WHAT IT TAKES TO BE A BIOMEDICAL EQUIPMENT TECHNICIAN?

If you are interested in becoming a biomedical equipment technician, you should have technical aptitude for working on a variety of electronic equipment. You must also be detail oriented, enjoy working with your hands, and have excellent troubleshooting skills. Stamina and patience are also important, and you must be able to see projects through to the finish. There are times when you may be stumped by a problem, but you need to persevere and follow through.

Although biomedical equipment technicians are trained to fix and service electronic equipment, they must also communicate and work with others, so people skills are crucial. "I emphasize 'people skills' as a virtual prerequisite for employment in this field," says Dennis. "In any typical workday, biomed techs may interact with people in an especially wide range of ethnic backgrounds, cultures, and educational levels. Additionally, the staff in health care settings is usually predominantly female. So on the first day of class, I frankly advise students that this is not a profession for bigotry, intolerance, or male chauvinism. Beyond that, we emphasize communication skills since biomeds must be able to speak and write reasonably well."

In addition, you must be adept at listening to others as they explain problems with equipment, and you need to be able to communicate clearly and tactfully when you are training people or correcting operator error.

HOW DO I BECOME A BIOMEDICAL EQUIPMENT TECHNICIAN?

Education

High School

It's never too early to start preparing for a biomedical equipment technician

(BMET) career. In high school, you should take mathematics (algebra and trigonometry) classes as well as science courses (including physics and chemistry). Shop classes can help you develop skills working with various tools, and if an electronics shop class is available, you should definitely enroll.

Computer science classes are helpful as well. As biomedical equipment becomes increasingly computerized, understanding how computers function is important. Health science classes will acquaint you with medical terminology and basic anatomy, both very important in the realm of the BMET. Not only must you understand the electronic equipment, but you must also know how the equipment affects or works with the patient.

If there is an opportunity to join an electronics club in your school or community, you should. Many high schools also participate in statewide or nationwide technical or science fairs, which give students an opportunity to build various objects and compete against other schools. These fairs are an excellent opportunity for you to gain some experience seeing projects through to the end, working with hand tools, and troubleshooting.

Postsecondary Training

Although a college degree is not absolutely mandatory to become a biomedical equipment technician, it is highly recommended, and most employers list a degree as a hiring requirement. Most technicians earn two-year associate degrees in biomedical technology. These two-year programs are available at both community colleges and technical schools. Only two institutions (Cincinnati State Technical and Community College, and Pennsylvania State University, New Kensington Campus) are accredited by the Technology Accreditation Commission for the Accreditation Board for Engineering and Technology (ABET). Training is also available through the armed forces.

A two-year degree in electronics is sometimes acceptable, but because biomedical technology is rather specialized, it is preferable to find a biomedical technology program.

Courses in biomedical technology programs can include mathematics, chemistry, applied physics, computer programming, medical terminology, digital and analog circuits, anatomy and physiology, advanced principles of electronics, and fundamentals of fluid power and electromechanical systems. "In college," says Myron Hartman, "math is the foundation of all technical classes. The BET program requires the student to take technical algebra, technical trigonometry, and technical calculus. Being proficient in math not only helps the student advance to the next higher level of math, but the math is used in almost all of the technical classes: electrical circuits 1 & 2, digital electronics, physics, chemistry, biology, biomedical classes, CAD, drafting, and engineering fundamentals." Myron also stresses the importance of English classes, as BET students will "be writing papers; reading textbooks; presenting speeches and technical presentations; communicating with students, faculty and coworkers during internships; preparing laboratory reports; and using computer software."

Biomedical equipment technicians must pursue continuing education throughout their careers in order to stay up to date with changing technology and new equipment. "As my students finish the second quarter of classwork," Dennis says, "I try to instill in them the idea of being responsible for their own continuing education. Employer-supported service schools are one thing, but techs should also read journals, take the occasional course in something pertinent to their career, and make an effort to attend meetings of their state or regional biomed society. My perception is that biomeds tend not to be good socializers, but mixing with their fellow techs can be very useful at several levels—especially for sounding out the job market. Biomed job openings are virtually never found in the classified ads of newspapers."

Certification or Licensing

The Board of Examiners for Biomedical Equipment Technicians, which is affiliated with the Association for the Advancement of Medical Instrumentation (AAMI), maintains certification programs for BMETs. The following categories are available: biomedical equipment technician, radiology equipment specialist, and clinical laboratory equipment specialist. "The AAMI certification is not required by most employers," says Dennis McMahon, "but I encourage students to make the effort to pass it within a year of finishing school. Being certified carries a certain weight when applying for positions, and a recent survey shows that certified techs are, on average, paid slightly better.

More importantly, certification conveys an attitude of professionalism that the biomed community needs to foster."

Internships and Volunteerships

Internships are an excellent way to gain experience, skills, and connections in the biomedical field. Internships are often required for students in associate degree programs and can lead to job opportunities after graduation. They are usually set up through the placement department and are without pay. Employers are fond of internships because it provides them a chance to teach aspiring technicians about the field. It is also a means to seek job candidates. Students in Penn State New Kensington's BET internship program work 400 hours in a hospital environment. "The internship program provides a structure for students to develop entry-level skills in the biomedical field, while gaining valuable work experience before graduation," Myron Hartman explains. "The program consists of biomedical hands-on experience in an actual work environment on medical equipment, with interns performing installations, service, and preventative maintenance inspections and hazard alert/recalls. The students also learn hospital operations by reviewing policy and procedures, attending specific meetings, observing surgical and clinical procedures, observing emergency generator testing, and participating in specific educational programs, such as infection control and general safety. The internship program aims to enable students to attain the following objectives: to acquire practical experience not available in a classroom setting; to increase the awareness of career demands; to identify skill strength and weaknesses; and to accumulate valid work experience before seeking permanent employment. On some occasions, internships lead to part-time, temporary, or full-time work. Feedback from graduates of the program all comment that the internship experience was one of the best classes in the BET program."

Volunteer opportunities in medical facilities are plentiful as well. Volunteering can give you some exposure to the industry and to the health care field in general.

Labor Unions

Union membership depends on the employer. There is no union specifically for biomedical equipment technicians, which means that technicians must usually join the union that represents the majority of the other health care workers in the facility. Some of the unions BMETs can join include the International Brotherhood of Electrical Workers and the International Union of Operating Engineers.

WHO WILL HIRE ME?

Approximately 29,000 biomedical equipment technicians are employed in the United States. Many technicians are employed by hospitals of all sizes. The federal government is another employer of BMETs, primarily through the Veterans Administration Hospitals and medical centers on military bases. Technicians working for manufacturers often special-

---

Advancement Possibilities

- *Biomedical engineers* design medical apparatus, including pacemakers, artificial organs, and ultrasonic imaging devices, by applying engineering principles.

- *Clinical engineers* design and evaluate biomedical systems and are involved with technology management.

- *Regional service managers* represent manufacturers or third-party companies. They supervise field offices and teams of technicians and may also develop customer relations and provide training to customers.

- *Customer service representatives* handle queries from customers about all aspects of the particular type of biomedical equipment their company sells.

---

ize in the repair of machinery. It is commonplace for manufacturing companies to provide maintenance agreements on new equipment, and biomedical equipment technicians are equipped to service the machinery. They may also install the equipment and train the operators or in-house technicians on its functions.

Independent service companies, or third-party companies, also service equipment. Hospitals that do not employ in-house biomedical equipment technicians may use the services of these third-party companies for repair, maintenance, and installation of equipment. Research and development departments within companies may also employ technicians to help test new equipment.

You might also consider becoming involved with local biomedical associations and attending the meetings to find out about what is happening in the biomedical community and to develop some relationships and connections.

The Internet may provide some leads on job openings. Many large hospitals, manufacturers, and health care organizations have job hotlines that announce new openings. These are often updated weekly. You might also send resumes and cover letters to all the facilities in the state you wish to live in to inquire about job possibilities.

Dennis offers the following advice to new graduates: "I encourage graduating students to be flexible with where they find job opportunities, and be realistic about beginning salary levels." He also advises graduates to consider options outside of traditional medical settings. "They may find that there are jobs for which biomed training is well suited, but have nothing to do with health care." A former tech at Dennis' company left to take a job working on the X-ray scanners used at airports.

WHERE CAN I GO FROM HERE?

After several years of experience and training, technicians employed in hospitals are promoted to higher-level positions. "Those in higher-level positions normally work on more complex systems," Myron Hartman explains, "as these systems require workers with advanced training and experience to understand, inspect, and service them. Working at the higher level positions also demands that the BMET be on-call for the evenings and weekends to answer and respond to emergency calls."

Technicians with advanced training and experience can become *BMET specialists*. "These workers," says Myron Hartman, "are highly trained and experienced, and normally earn the highest salaries. Technicians typically specialize in imaging (X-ray, computerized tomography scanners, magnetic resonance imaging, nuclear medicine, or ultrasound), surgical services, or computers/networking/information. Other career routes include going into management positions and becoming a supervisor, manager, or director of a clinical engineering department. These positions have a shift in responsibilities from technical to management. These types of technicians are now more focused on regulatory and standard compliance, budgets, personnel issues, department and hospital goals, and policy and procedure compliance. Training and education in business or management is a plus if someone desires to go into supervision."

With a four-year degree in biomedical engineering, technicians may become *biomedical* or *clinical engineers* and assist in the research and design of new equipment and processes. Clinical engineers are engineers who assess and repair biomedical systems and may be involved in technology management. They are more concerned with the big picture than with individual pieces of equipment. Biomedical engineers, on the other hand, design medical equipment and instruments by applying engineering principles.

Biomedical equipment technicians who enter the industry as field service technicians with manufacturers or third-party companies can move into regional service management positions. *Regional service managers* supervise biomedical equipment technicians and other staff and may oversee a number of field offices or service centers. Managers may also provide training to customers and solicit new clients.

Dennis McMahon says that he plans to retire in about five years. "I am in that upper-50s demographic group that will be out of the active market in about five years. But just as a hypothetical, if I were in my 40s and were charting a course for the last half of my career, I'd strive to get additional specialty training in order to allow more flexibility in compensation and type of employer. An example is taking classes in networking and information systems, and working for a manufacturer of image-guided surgical systems."

WHAT ARE THE SALARY RANGES?

Salaries for biomedical equipment technicians vary in different institutions and localities and according to the experience, training, certification, and type of work done by the technician. According to the U.S. Department of Labor, medical equipment repairers had median earnings of

Related Jobs

- biomedical engineers
- cardiovascular technologists
- communications equipment technicians
- computer and office machine service technicians
- diagnostic medical sonographers
- dialysis technicians
- electrical and electronics engineers
- electroneurodiagnostic technologists
- electronics engineering technicians
- medical laboratory technicians
- microelectronics technicians
- radiologic technologists
- respiratory therapists and technicians
- wireless service technicians

$38,590 in 2004. Salaries ranged from less than $22,630 to $60,050 or more.

According to *24x7*, a publication for health care technical service and support professionals, biomedical technicians earned an average base salary of $51,289 in 2005. Additionally, the magazine reports that technicians employed in all medical specialties who were certified earned average base salaries of $58,164, while those who were not certified earned only $54,387 annually.

Biomedical equipment technicians usually receive generous benefits packages with medical benefits, pension plans, and more. Employers may also finance continuing education courses and seminars.

WHAT IS THE JOB OUTLOOK?

The *Occupational Outlook Handbook* indicates that jobs for biomedical equipment technicians will grow about as fast as the average. Technological advances will affect the health care industry, and qualified biomedical equipment technicians will be needed to install, maintain, and repair equipment, as well as train operators on proper usage and care. "There will always be technology applied to health care delivery," says Dennis, "and the technology will continue to evolve. There is equipment in use today that was almost considered science fiction 30 years ago. Thirty years from now, it is hard to imagine what will be in use, but there will be a need for personnel to maintain it and repair it." In the future, equipment will rely more heavily on microprocessors and computers, which will also create a need for skilled technicians. New instruments and machines are developed and manufactured on a regular basis, and technicians are qualified to evaluate, test, and make recommendations from both the purchasing end and the design end.

Myron Hartman also feels that employment is strong for biomedical equipment technicians. "I think the employment opportunity is the best it has ever been," he says. "With only two ABET-accredited schools in the nation and fewer BET programs in general, there are less qualified people entering the profession. Individuals who started in the field in the late '70s are approaching retirement age, with some advancing to management and other related positions. Some hospitals have hired individuals with electronics or computer science degrees, but these individuals do not have the necessary fundamentals to be proficient as a BMET. Since I have been at Penn State, our employment placement is close to 100 percent. Graduates make good starting salaries and advancement normally happens within a year or so after employment."

Myron says that one of the biggest problems in getting more people interested in the field is that very few know it exists. "Guidance counselors, high school teachers, and the public in general are not even aware of the profession," he says. "Most people discover the program through a neighbor or relative who works in the field. But for those who do discover it, it is a very rewarding career. If you have good people skills, a good attitude, are open to relocation, and have passing grades and fairly good technical skills, you will get a job in this profession."

The state of health care may influence the outlook for biomedical equipment technicians. As the trend toward health maintenance organizations (HMOs) increases, medical facilities will be persuaded to adopt cost-cutting measures. Biomedical equipment technicians will therefore be in demand to keep the existing equipment in top working condition.

Additionally, Dennis points out that the aging of the baby boomer generation will also ensure increased demand for medical services as a result of technicians in their 50s and 60s retiring. "In the latest salary survey," says Dennis, "I noticed that 61 percent of the responding biomeds are over 50 years old. We can reasonably expect that over the next 15 years, there will be a brisk level of retirement, creating job openings by natural attrition."

Diagnostic Medical Sonographers

SUMMARY

Definition
Diagnostic medical sonographers use advanced medical technology, in the form of high-frequency sound waves, to produce images of the internal body structures for analysis by radiologists and other physicians.

Alternative Job Title
Ultrasound technologists

Salary Range
$38,620 to $53,650 to $73,600+

Educational Requirements
Associate degree, hospital certificate program, or bachelor's degree

Certification or Licensing
Required (certification)
Required by certain states (licensing)

Outlook
Much faster than the average

High School Subjects
Anatomy and physiology
Biology
Computer science
Health
Mathematics

Personal Skills
Helping people: physical/ health medicine
Science

The young expectant mother waits on an examination table, her forehead creased with lines. It seems like weeks since she last felt the sharp kick of her baby from within her body. She is worried that something has gone wrong with the development of her child.

The diagnostic medical sonographer (DMS) maintains a steady dialogue with the frightened woman in order to distract her from her anxiety; she calms her patient with gentle humor as she coats her stomach with ultrasound gel. She then explains the procedure and positions the woman in order to assure optimum scanning.

Using a device called a transducer, the sonographer directs high-frequency sound waves toward the unborn baby. These waves will reflect off the body tissue to form a two-dimensional, real-time image on a video monitor.

The DMS is careful to observe the screen as she moves the transducer, aware of the need for a high-quality ultrasound image.

An image of a baby, a healthy boy, appears. The sonographer quickly points to the baby's beating heart on the monitor. She also points out the baby's head and other body parts; and the mother is overwhelmed with happiness and relief.

The DMS is extremely happy for the young woman, yet also knows there is a job to complete. She finishes recording the images of the baby and prepares the film to be taken to a physician for further analysis. This high degree of professionalism, combined with compassion, allows diagnostic medical sonographers to be prepared and able to do their jobs in the event of good news, as with the young mother, or bad news. The image of another young mother whose baby girl did not survive still lingers in her memory.

The sonographer wishes the young woman well and readies her equipment for the next patient. In the course of her day she will complete procedures that test for cysts, abdominal tumors, and impeded function of blood vessels and heart valves.

WHAT DOES A DIAGNOSTIC MEDICAL SONOGRAPHER DO?

Diagnostic medical sonographers (DMSs), sometimes known as *ultrasound technologists,* or simply *sonographers,* use high-frequency sound waves, which are an offshoot of World War II SONAR technology, to produce images of the internal body. A picture is obtained when these sound waves bounce off internal structures, becoming echoes that are then displayed as two-dimensional gray images on a video screen. The recorded images are used by a physician in diagnosing disease and in studying the malfunction of organs.

Diagnostic medical sonographers, working under the supervision of a qualified physician, are responsible for the selection and the setup of the proper ultrasound equipment for each specific examination. They also explain the procedure to the patient, record any additional information that may help in the diagnosis, and help the patient into the proper physical position so the test may begin.

When the patient is properly aligned, the sonographer applies ultrasound gel to the specific test area. He or she is responsible for selecting the transducer and adjusting controls in relation to the depth of field, organ or structure examined, and other factors. The sonographer physically moves the transducer, a microphone-shaped device that sends high-frequency sound waves into the area to be imaged. At the same time, the sonographer watches the video monitor to be sure that a quality ultrasonic image is being produced. The sonographer must also be aware of subtle differences between healthy and diseased areas in order to be able to record the correct image.

Once the target area is located and a quality image appears consistently on screen, the sonographer then activates the equipment that begins to record images on magnetic tape, a computer disc, strip printout, radiographic or video paper film, or videotape. The sonographer is responsible for filming individual views or sequences of real-time images in affected areas. When a procedure is completed, the sonographer removes the film and prepares it for analysis by a specially

Lingo to Learn

Doppler A stethoscope-like instrument that is used to measure blood-flow velocity.

megahertz The degree of strength for a sound wave in an ultrasound procedure.

M mode A reading that determines the fetal heart rate.

sonography A diagnostic procedure that uses sound waves, instead of radiation, to create an image of the human body.

transducer A technologist-controlled device that directs high-frequency sound waves to a specific body part in order to create a two-dimensional moving image for analysis.

trained physician. The sonographer may also be asked to discuss the test with a supervisor or attending physician.

In addition to diagnostic procedures, sonographers must also maintain patient data relating to each test, and check and adjust their equipment to ensure that readings are accurate. They may also, after considerable experience, have a role in preparing work schedules and evaluating potential equipment purchases.

WHAT IS IT LIKE TO BE A DIAGNOSTIC MEDICAL SONOGRAPHER?

Terry Ciez is the program coordinator of the Diagnostic Medical Imaging Sonography and Vascular Programs at the College of DuPage in Glen Ellyn, Illinois. She has worked at the college for seven years and as a diagnostic medical sonographer for 32 years. "I started my medical career 35 years ago when I entered the radiology program at Moraine Valley Community College," she recalls. "I finished the program, and then continued on at Northwestern University in the nuclear medicine program. While I was in the nuclear medicine program, sonography had just been introduced. The hospital wasn't sure where to place sonography, so the machine was placed in the nuclear medicine department. I was asked if I would like to learn the sonography portion. At the time, not even the radiologists knew how to interpret or scan, so we kind of all learned together hands-on. In the morning I would complete nuclear medicine scans, and in the afternoon I would do all of their ultrasound exams."

After working in a hospital environment for a number of years, Terrie began working as a product manager in nuclear medicine and professional education, as well as ultrasound. "I traveled worldwide," she recalls, "teaching various hospitals and technologists how to perform ultrasound exams, as well as setting up educational programs. After that, I started my own mobile ultrasound business, B & C Imaging Consultants, which I still have, where we travel to doctor's offices to perform ultrasound exams on patients. Concurrently, I also teach the general sonography program at the College of DuPage."

Terrie typically divides her workday between performing ultrasound examinations via her mobile ultrasound busi-

To Be a Successful Diagnostic Medical Sonographer, You Should . . .

- have good communication skills, oral and written

- have patience for sometimes monotonous or repetitious procedures

- enjoy helping and working with people as part of a team

- be technically adept and detail-oriented

- have a compassionate nature

terminology. They must have a superior understanding of human physiology, combined with an artistic approach in order to visualize human anatomy.

DMSs must also have good communication skills to understand and implement physicians' orders, and also to instruct and guide patients into the proper position.

Like other members of the diagnostic field, DMSs must learn to be objective and unemotional in order to accomplish their duties. DMSs must also possess good people skills such as compassion, patience, kindness, and empathy in order to help very ill, scared, young, or very old patients understand and complete a procedure.

ness and her work as program coordinator at the College of DuPage. "In the mornings," she says, "I will scan in a doctor's office and perform various obstetrical exams for the patients and prepare them to be read by a radiologist. I spend afternoons and evenings at the college coordinating and teaching our students the various aspects of general sonography in obstetrics, gynecology, abdominal, and superficial structures (which entails breast, scrotum, and thyroid). It's a pretty full day, five days a week."

DO I HAVE WHAT IT TAKES TO BE A DIAGNOSTIC MEDICAL SONOGRAPHER?

DMSs should be technically adept and possess a thorough knowledge of medical

Advancement Possibilities

- *Chief technologists and administrators* are sonographers who, as a result of advanced education and experience, have risen to supervisory positions in hospitals and other medical settings.

- *Sonography instructors* teach in technical programs, teaching hospitals, and university settings.

- *Sales representatives* for ultrasonic equipment sell electronic devices that clean, test, or process materials by means of high-frequency sound waves, such as disintegrators for cleaning surgical instruments, electronic guns for bonding plastics, and sonic devices for detecting flaws in metals, cutting steel and diamonds, and separating fossils from rocks.

Although diagnostic sonography does not involve harmful radiation, DMSs should be aware that they will be exposed to sick people who might carry communicable diseases. Universal standards do exist to ensure safety for both patient and technologist. The only hazardous material that sonographers are exposed to is waste from invasive procedures.

DMSs can assure continuing safety by keeping updated on current hazardous waste disposal methods and being diligent in applying universal safety standards to every procedure.

HOW DO I BECOME A DIAGNOSTIC MEDICAL SONOGRAPHER?

Education

High School

Students intent on a career in diagnostic medical sonography should take courses in biology, physics, anatomy and physiology, mathematics, speech, and technical writing. Students still in high school should take four years of science, when possible, especially chemistry, since it is a main component of the state boards that grant licensure.

Postsecondary Training

Instruction in diagnostic medical sonography is offered at technical schools, colleges, and universities in the form of four-year bachelor's programs, two-year associate programs, in teaching hospitals in the form of a two-year hospital certificate, and also in the armed forces. Students in these programs take general education courses, as well as learn about the field via hands-on training. "Along with teaching courses," Terrie says, "our program has hands-on courses in the classroom where the students actually scan one another in order to learn how to identify normal structures and anatomy and then be able to understand the pathology of various organs. This allows them to understand what they are seeing and convey this information to the radiologist."

Terrie encourages prospective students to thoroughly check school accreditation before investing their time and money. "It's important that students attend an accredited program," she says. "When a college is not accredited, that means that when a student finishes the program, they cannot take their registry with the American Registry of Diagnostic Medical Sonographers. If you are not registered, many hospitals and medical offices will not hire you." The Commission on Accreditation for Allied Health Education Programs (http://www.caahep.org) accredits sonography education programs. More than 130 such programs exist in the United States.

Certification and Licensing

All medical employers of DMSs require certification by the American Registry of Diagnostic Medical Sonographers (ARDMS). After completion of educational requirements, DMSs must register with ARDMS and take and pass the National Boards to obtain their license. The ARDMS administers examinations and awards credentials in diagnostic medical sonography, diagnostic cardiac sonography, and vascular technology. Licensing requirements may exist at the state level also, although requirements vary from state to state.

Internships and Volunteerships

Students in sonography programs are typically required to participate in clinical rotations, which allow them to gain experience in hospital and other medical

Ultrasonics

Ultrasonics is the branch of physics and engineering dealing with high-frequency sound waves. The waves are produced by objects vibrating more than 20,000 times a second, creating sound that is beyond the range of human hearing—ultrasound.

Ultrasonic vibrations may be created electronically by passing alternating current through a quartz or ceramic crystal; mechanically, with special sirens; or magnetically, by the action of an alternating magnetic field on a hollow metal rod.

Pierre Curie discovered how to produce ultrasonic vibrations in 1890. By World War II their first practical application—the detection of submarines underwater—had been developed (i.e., sonar).

Today ultrasonic waves have many important applications. In addition to the medical imaging uses discussed in this chapter, ultrasonic energy is also used in medicine to heat deep tissues. The method has been used to treat arthritis, bursitis, muscular dystrophy, and other diseases. High-energy ultrasonic waves can also be focused into a pinpoint "scalpel" for bloodless brain surgery.

In dentistry, ultrasonic devices are sometimes used to remove calcium deposits from the surface of teeth.

Ultrasonic vibrations in a liquid cause millions of bubbles to form and collapse thousands of times a second. This process, called cavitation, blasts clean the surface of objects immersed in the liquid. Applications of this process include sterilization of surgical instruments and the scouring of precision metal parts. Diamonds, tungsten carbide, and tool steel are readily carved and drilled by ultrasonic techniques. The material to be machined is fixed in place and the cutting tool is lowered until it is in contact with the surface. Then a liquid abrasive is poured over the material in a steady stream. The tool vibrates at an ultrasonic frequency and drives tiny particles of the abrasive against the material with tremendous impact. This bombardment, together with cavitation, grinds an exact counterpart of the tool face into the material being machined. Odd-shaped cuts not possible with other methods can be made.

Sound waves beamed into solid materials will not readily cross air barriers such as cracks. When a crack or other defect is encountered, the sound waves are reflected to a measuring instrument. This form of inspection has replaced the use of X-rays in many industries.

Ultrasound is used in some types of burglar alarms and remote-control television tuners. It is also sometimes used in welding and soldering metals, mixing liquids, and dyeing and bleaching textiles.

settings. "Three days a week," Terrie says, "students in our program rotate into a hospital and have the opportunity to perform scans on patients under the guidance of a registered technologist and radiologist. These clinical rotations allow students to acquire and improve their hands-on imaging skills."

Although no one except a licensed DMS may actually work in the field, experience and insight may be gained from dialogue with a DMS, visiting a job site, or for those still in high school, arranging informational exchanges between student groups and a local employer of diagnostic medical sonographers. Another possibility for experience is to speak with a teacher at an accredited ultrasound program.

WHO WILL HIRE ME?

Approximately 42,000 diagnostic medical sonographers are employed in the United States. Hospitals are the main employers of sonographers. Career opportunities also exist in health maintenance organizations (HMOs), private physicians' offices, imaging centers, mobile imaging clinics, clinical research labs, educational institutions, and industry. They may also work in departments of cardiology, radiology, obstetrics, and vascular surgery

Registered technologists should seek out the publications of professional organizations, such as the Society of Diagnostic Medical Sonography, which maintains a list of job openings (see the "Look to the Pros" chapter in this book). Other avenues include employment agencies specializing in the health care field, "headhunters," or

direct application to the personnel officers of potential health care employers.

Rural areas and small towns may offer the best employment opportunities for those willing to relocate and accept lower wages and compensation as compared to jobs in larger cities.

WHERE CAN I GO FROM HERE?

There are many avenues of advancement open to experienced DMSs, yet technologists and prospective students should be aware that advancement can only occur through further education. Those with a bachelor's degree or higher stand the best chance for promotion or advancement. Advanced education can be obtained through technical programs, colleges and universities, teaching hospitals, and sometimes through in-house retraining. Further education will allow DMSs to become certified in nuclear medicine technology, radiation therapy, magnetic resonance imaging, CT scan, computer tomography, or special procedures. Terrie just completed her master's degree in health science administration at the University of St. Francis, and plans to pursue a Ph.D. in health care. "In five years," she predicts, "I would love being in my same position and being able to continue to teach students to be the best sonographers in their field, because one day, I will probably be their patient, and I want to ensure that all patients have a good, quality exam."

With considerable experience, DMSs, such as Terrie, can rise to teaching positions in sonography education programs, or train other technologists in-house or at another location. Other DMSs may become involved in the sales and marketing aspect of their profession, working as equipment demonstrators and instructors for the medical industry. In a hospital setting, DMSs with advanced degrees can become clinical supervisors, administrators, or assume other managerial positions.

WHAT ARE THE SALARY RANGES?

According to the U.S. Department of Labor, diagnostic medical sonographers earned a median annual income of $53,650 in 2004. The lowest paid 10 percent of this group, which included those just beginning in the field, made $38,620 or less. The highest paid 10 percent, which included those with experience and managerial duties, earned $73,600 or more annually.

Hospital DMSs and those employed in outpatient care centers earn less on average than those technologists employed by HMOs, private physicians' offices, and medical and diagnostic laboratories, and other employers. As always, pay scales and compensation vary based on education level, experience and responsibilities, and location of employers, with urban employers offering more financial compensation than rural or small town employers. Beyond base salaries, sonographers can expect to enjoy many fringe benefits, including paid vacation, sick and personal days, and health and dental insurance.

Related Jobs

- biomedical equipment technicians
- cardiovascular technologists
- dialysis technicians
- electroneurodiagnostic technologists
- medical assistants
- medical laboratory technicians
- ophthalmic laboratory technicians
- optics technicians
- orthotic and prosthetic technicians
- radiologic technologists
- respiratory therapists and technicians

WHAT IS THE JOB OUTLOOK?

According to the U.S. Department of Labor, employment of diagnostic medical sonographers should grow much faster than the average. One reason for this growth is that sonography is a safe, non-radioactive imaging process. In addition, sonography has proved successful in detecting life-threatening diseases and in analyzing previously nonimageable internal organs.

"The employment outlook for sonography is wonderful," Terrie says. "Because there are so many specialties, there is a higher need for trained technologists. Here at the College of DuPage, we train students in four: the abdomen, superficial structures, obstetrics/gynecology, and general applications of physics. Once they acquire these skills they can branch into other specialties, such as vascular, echocardiography, neurology, or ophthalmology."

Although not as big as the radiology field, diagnostic sonography offers excellent prospects. Ultrasound technology will enjoy even more widespread use, especially in the expanding fields of obstetrics/gynecology and cardiology. Demand for qualified DMSs exceeds the supply in some areas of the country, especially in rural areas and small towns. Those who are flexible about pay scales and compensation will find ready employment in these areas.

Those interested in the diagnostic field should be aware of potential roadblocks to future employment. The health care industry currently is in a state of great potential change as the government and public debate future health care policy and the role of third-party payers in the system. Some procedures may not be readily used due to their cost to insurance companies and the government. Job opportunities and growth may be limited as a result.

Hospitals will also continue to downsize, causing some procedures to be done on weekends, nights, or on an outpatient basis. Future DMSs should be aware of the growth of imaging centers, HMOs, and physicians' offices as significant employers of their profession. These employers will compete with hospitals for the most qualified DMSs.

Prospective sonographers need to be aware that competition exists for good jobs. Those with advanced education, experience, and certification in other specialized areas such as CT scan, mammography, radiation therapy, nuclear medicine technology, and other fields stand to prosper in future job markets.

Genetic Counselors

SUMMARY

Definition
Genetic counselors are health care professionals who work with individuals who may be at risk for a variety of inherited conditions or who have family members with birth defects or genetic disorders.

Alternative Job Titles
None

Salary Range
$33,000 to $53,777 to $97,000

Educational Requirements
Master's degree

Certification or Licensing
Recommended

Employment Outlook
Much faster than the average

High School Subjects
Anatomy and physiology

Biology
Health
Mathematics
Science

Personal Interests
Helping people: emotionally
Helping people: physical health/medicine
Psychology
Science

"When a pregnancy has been found to have multiple problems," says genetic counselor Elizabeth Leeth, "parents want answers that are sometimes impossible to give. I have had a couple of cases in which we did testing for chromosome abnormalities that came back normal. This was upsetting to the parents to not have a cause. In one, the baby died and we were not sure of the reason. But through the examination of the baby, certain abnormalities were identified. I urged them to have an autopsy (which, of course, is hard to think about at such a time). The results of the autopsy helped me to pinpoint a diagnosis, which has then allowed me to give them an accurate recurrence risk. Although it was not good news, it gave them some concrete information. This family is currently not cared for by our institution due to insurance changes; however, they call me at every pregnancy, and after the birth of a healthy son, have sent me pictures and holiday cards thanking me for my support and information."

WHAT DOES A GENETIC COUNSELOR DO?

Genetic counselors translate technical information about inherited health disorders into language that can be understood by the average person. They explain health disorders, the available options for testing for or treatment of these disorders, and the risks associated with each option. They also help patients come to terms with the emotional and psychological aspects of having an inherited disorder or disease.

Expectant parents are among the many families who may benefit from genetic counseling. Other couples who already have one child with an inherited disorder or whose families have a history of an inherited disorder may want information about the probability of having another child with that disorder. Individuals whose families have a history of inherited disease, such as Huntington's disease or muscular dystrophy, may want to know whether they have inherited the genes that give rise to these diseases. Individuals whose families have a high incidence of cancer may want to find out whether they have an inherited susceptibility to the disease. Members of specific geographic or ethnic groups in which a genetic disorder is common may want to determine what their risk is for developing the disorder.

When an individual schedules an appointment, the genetic counselor usually asks the patient to gather as much specific information about the past two generations of his or her family as possible. The counselor may ask for physicians' records, photographs, and anecdotal information. If a patient is concerned about inherited cancer, for instance, the physician wants to know how frequently the disease has occurred in the family, what types of cancer occurred, and at

what age family members developed the disease. All of this information provides the genetic counselor with important clues about the patient's genetic probability of inheriting a disease.

Before going any further, the genetic counselor explains the risks, benefits, and limitations of pursuing genetic testing. Some genetic testing presents physical risks, like those associated with amniocentesis. Others present emotional and psychological risks. If a patient discovers, for instance, that he or she has inherited the genes for Huntington's disease, how will he or she cope with knowing that this disease will develop at some later time? What if a patient wants to obtain genetic information about his or her family, but other siblings do not want this information and refuse to participate in its discovery? Genetic counselors want patients to be aware of and prepared for these situations. Genetic counselors also inform patients that genetic testing may threaten their insurability. If an insurance company discovers that a patient has inherited a genetic susceptibility for cancer, for example, that person may have a very difficult time getting coverage or may be charged higher premiums than individuals who do not have this genetic trait.

If a patient decides to proceed with testing, the genetic counselor interprets the test results, discusses treatment options, and explains the risks, both physical and emotional, associated with the various treatment options. Throughout the counseling process, the genetic counselor must remain supportive of the patient's choices.

Lingo to Learn

amniocentesis Sampling of the amniotic fluid contained in the uterus during pregnancy.

chorionic villus sampling An invasive test that takes a biopsy of the placenta to detect chromosome abnormalities such as Down syndrome. The test also can be used for DNA and biochemical testing.

chromosomes Threadlike structures of nucleic acids and protein that carry genes.

Down syndrome A chromosome disorder that results in abnormal physical development. Many people with this condition are mildly retarded.

first trimester screening A diagnostic test that determines the risk for Down syndrome by testing the levels of certain chemicals in a pregnant woman's blood.

genes The units of heredity that are transmitted from parents to offspring and control or determine a single characteristic in the offspring.

Huntington's disease A hereditary disease that causes progressive brain-cell degeneration, resulting in spasmodic body movements and mental confusion.

maternal serum screening A diagnostic test that that determines the risk for open neural tube defect, Down syndrome, or trisomy 18 by testing the levels of certain proteins in a pregnant woman's blood.

muscular dystrophy A group of hereditary diseases characterized by the wasting away of muscles.

pharmacogenetics The study of how genetic differences affect patients' responses to medications.

teratogens Agents that cause malformation in developing embryos.

ultrasonography The process of creating an ultrasound image of structures deep within the body. Ultrasound images can be used for fetal monitoring and to show fetal development.

In addition to their counseling responsibilities, genetic counselors often assume administrative or teaching responsibilities. They also discuss test results with laboratory technicians and answer physicians' questions. Some supervise graduate students who are training to become genetic counselors. Because the available genetic information is increasing so rapidly, all genetic counselors must read extensively and attend conferences to learn about new developments in genetic research. Many also strive to educate the public and physicians about the availability of genetic counseling.

WHAT IS IT LIKE TO BE A GENETIC COUNSELOR?

Elizabeth Leeth is a genetic counselor at Evanston Northwestern Healthcare (EHN) in Evanston, Illinois. She has worked in the field for more than 12 years—all at ENH. Elizabeth works in the Fetal Diagnostic Center doing prenatal genetics. "When I first started here," she recalls, "I worked with one other genetic counselor. Currently, there are six genetic counselors employed as prenatal counselors at ENH."

Over the past two years, Elizabeth has moved into an administrative role as the assistant manager of fetal diagnostics. "This involves the supervision of the secretarial staff, genetic counselors, and administrative responsibilities for the registered nurses and ultrasound technicians," she explains. "Our Fetal Diagnostic Center sees approximately 10,000 ultrasounds per year. The genetic counselors see approximately 2,500 cases a year. These include pre-procedure counseling for amniocentesis and chorionic villus sampling, first trimester Down syndrome screening patients (a screen involving ultrasound and a blood test to determine a risk factor for Down syndrome), abnormal ultrasound patients [those in which the fetus has an abnormality (i.e., a heart defect, missing kidneys, etc.)], patients who have babies born with birth defects (when in the infant special care unit), pre-conception or early pregnancy counseling for family history issues, carrier screening for cystic fibrosis, and an Ashkenazi Jewish panel."

Elizabeth currently does not see as many patients as she did prior to moving into administration. "This is both bad and good," she reflects. "Bad, because I very much enjoy the interaction and possible impact that a genetic counselor can have

with families through the support and information we provide. Good, because this can be an emotionally taxing job at times due to the sharing of tragic experiences with these families. Also, being involved in the administrative side of the hospital has also given me the opportunity to educate health care workers outside of fetal diagnostics/genetics about the importance of genetic counseling in the health care field in general. This has been important, as many people, even in health care fields, are not sure as to what genetic counselors offer."

"Back when," Elizabeth says, "a normal day involved taking phone calls regarding questions about family history, abnormal screen results, testing/screening options, and risk factors involved. Depending on the call, research may be required, which now involves computer literature searches, database searches, and possible e-mails/phone calls to labs to get detailed information and availability. At any point I could be called to see a patient who has had an ultrasound with an abnormality identified in the fetus. This may have been suspected or has come out of the blue. These meetings involve discussing the understanding of what the physician has told them about the problem (let's say a heart defect), what could be the causes, what other testing may help to identify the cause, and also other possible problems that may be there (i.e., doing an amniocentesis and finding out it may be Down syndrome), offering resources and support, and arranging follow-up referrals or appointments (i.e., a meeting with a neonatologist or surgeon). Once that patient has left, there may then be an appointment for an Ashkenazi Jewish Panel, which involves discussing with an individual or couple the diseases for which someone with Jewish descent may be at risk to pass on to their children, what the inheritance patterns are, what the actual risks are, and what the screening will offer them. This would be followed up by a letter to the referring physician with results. If this were a Wednesday, we would attend the weekly perinatal conference, during which patients are presented and an educational presentation is given. The genetic counselors are responsible for leading this once a month.

"Currently, my day may involve any of these things or not. I now make sure that schedules are correct, patients are scheduled for appropriate appointments, any emergent situations are handled, technical issues (electronic patient chart issues, orders, reports, etc.) are addressed, and complaints are dealt with. All the fun stuff!"

In addition to managing genetic counselors and working as a genetic counselor, Elizabeth also serves as an instructor for a three-quarter course at Northwestern University's Graduate Program in Genetic Counseling, which meets three times a week. "I give lectures on diverse topics and coordinate guest lecturers and exams," she explains. "During the summer and some of the year, the other genetic counselors and I supervise students in their clinical rotations."

Christina Laning has worked as a prenatal genetic counselor at the University of Illinois-Chicago (UIC) Medical Center, Division of Maternal Fetal Medicine, since 2005. "I am a full-time genetic counselor who works directly with one other genetic counselor and six maternal fetal medicine physicians," she says. "Throughout high school and my undergraduate education, I was planning to attend medical school after graduating from college. I was most interested in the OB/GYN and reproductive endocrinology/infertility specialties. During my last year as an undergrad, I decided that a career as a physician was not for me, so I decided to investigate other opportunities in my same interest area, and that is when I discovered the field of genetic counseling. For me, it is the perfect balance of science and psychosocial counseling, and as a prenatal counselor, I am able to fulfill my interests in the OB/GYN field."

To Be a Successful Genetic Counselor, You Should . . .

- enjoy both science and working with people
- know your own biases and be nonjudgmental
- enjoy reading, learning, and working with developing technology
- be able to work in stressful, emotional situations
- enjoy helping people

Christina's practice includes all aspects of prenatal genetic counseling including providing information, risk assessment, genetic screening/testing, proper follow-up, and support for at-risk couples. Her other responsibilities include coordinating the UIC Perinatal Loss Clinic, resident/fellow and genetic counseling student education, and a weekly offsite prenatal clinic.

DO I HAVE WHAT IT TAKES TO BE A GENETIC COUNSELOR?

Genetic counselors wear two hats: they are scientists, and they are counselors. As scientists, genetic counselors must be able to think critically. They must be intellectually curious and read constantly to stay abreast of the ever-changing information in this field. As counselors, they regularly interact with people who may be undergoing the most difficult and painful experiences in their lives. Genetic counselors must be compassionate, and they must be able to convey complex information clearly and concisely. Genetic counselors regularly encounter tragic situations. They must be able to deliver unpleasant news gently, but directly. Helping families cope with frightening information and painful decisions can be extremely stressful.

HOW DO I BECOME A GENETIC COUNSELOR?
Education
Elizabeth Leeth learned about genetic counseling as a senior in high school and found it very interesting. "However," she recalls, "at that time, only two schools offered training, and the job market was small; I therefore did not think it was a feasible/reasonable career choice." Instead, Elizabeth became a science teacher and taught biology and chemistry in Indiana for five years. "The summer prior to my fifth year in teaching," she says, "I attended a five-week class sponsored by the Indiana Science Teachers Association, held at Indiana University, that was designed to update science teachers in subjects of genetics, immunology, and molecular biology. After speaking with the genetics professor about my special interest in genetics, he informed me that the medical school was going to offer a new degree in genetic counseling. I visited the genetics clinic in Indianapolis that fall, applied, and here I am. I was surprised to be accepted as I had been out of school for several years, but was very excited and remain extremely happy with that move."

High School
If you are interested in this career, you should begin by taking college preparatory courses in high school. Such classes as biology, physiology, chemistry, and statistics will help you determine your aptitude in these areas as well as prepare you for college. Since counseling skills are as important to the performance of this job as understanding genetics, you will also benefit from classes in sociology and psychology. English classes will help you develop your written communication skills, and speech classes will help you gain confidence in speaking.

Postsecondary Training

Getting your bachelor's degree is the next step to becoming a genetic counselor. Although no specific major is required, students entering this field typically have a degree in biologic science, social science, or a related field. Elizabeth Leeth earned a teaching degree in biology, with a chemistry minor, from Purdue University. Christina Laning earned a bachelor's of science in psychology and pre-medicine at the University of Michigan. Important college courses to take include general biology, developmental biology, genetics, chemistry, and statistics and probability. Other helpful courses include psychology, English, and ethics.

Following college, you must complete a master's degree. At present, more than 25 graduate schools offer programs in genetic counseling in the United States. To obtain a list of these programs and contact information, visit the American Board of Genetic Counseling's Web site, http://www.abgc.net. Elizabeth Leeth earned her master's of science in medical genetics from Indiana University/Purdue University of Indianapolis. Christina Laning earned a master's of science in genetic counseling from the University of South Carolina School of Medicine. Graduate school studies in genetic counseling typically include classes in client-centered counseling, issues in clinical genetics, medical genetics, biochemistry, human anatomy and physiology, and clinical medicine. All programs require field experience in clinical settings.

Certification or Licensing

Licensing is not required for genetic counselors. Certification is also not required, although it is highly recommended. Most employers will expect a genetic counselor to be certified. The American Board of Genetic Counseling (ABGC) offers certification in the United States through an exam offered every two years. Candidates must successfully complete both the general and specialty certification examination. In addition, they must have a graduate degree in genetic counseling, clinical experience in an ABGC-approved training site or sites, and a logbook of 50 supervised cases. The ABGC reports that 72 to 74 percent of candidates taking the test pass it successfully.

Internships and Volunteerships

Most schools require that students pursuing a degree in genetic counseling complete an internship. Internships provide students with hands-on work experience and the opportunity to network and gain a deeper understanding of the work of genetic counselors. Interns might work at university medical centers, local hospitals, diagnostic laboratories, or with physicians in private practice. Depending on their location, students might also find internships with government organizations such as the National Cancer Institute, the National Human Genome Research Institute, and the National Institutes of Health.

Volunteer experience is also extremely useful to individuals considering a genetic counseling career. Although experience in a medical setting is ideal, volunteer opportunities exist in many settings, such as at nursing homes, private clinics, and programs for people with disabilities. By exposing yourself to working with a wide variety of people with different needs and backgrounds, you may develop communication skills, problem-solving strategies, insight, and compassion.

WHO WILL HIRE ME?

In its biannual survey of members in 2004, the National Society of Genetic Councelors (NSGC) found that 41 percent of genetic counselors are employed by university medical centers. That number is slowly decreasing though, as private and public hospitals, health maintenance organizations (HMOs), diagnostic laboratories, and physicians in private practice are hiring more genetic counselors. Only 1 percent work in their own private practices, independent of a physician. Data published by the NSGC suggests that an increasing number of genetic counselors are working in genetic research.

WHERE CAN I GO FROM HERE?

Genetic counselors can advance by assuming teaching and administrative responsibilities. Research opportunities are available for individuals who earn a doctoral degree. Experts estimate that the available genetic information doubles every 18 months. As scientists and doctors learn to use the information provided by the mapping of the human genome, even more information will be available. Professionals in this field are constantly

learning, which may explain why 89 percent of genetic counselors describe themselves as "satisfied" with their careers, according to the NSGC.

WHAT ARE THE SALARY RANGES?

According to the NSGC 2004 survey of members, genetic counselors with a master's degree working full time received a mean salary of $53,377. Entry-level salaries were as low as $33,000, and genetic counselors with significant experience may earn as much as $97,000.

The same study indicated that, except at the highest levels, genetic counselors who are employed by the private sector, such as HMOs or private hospitals, generally are paid more than those who work for university medical centers or public

Related Jobs

- alcohol and drug abuse counselors
- biochemists
- biologists
- biomedical engineers
- genetic scientists
- human services workers
- medical geneticists
- medical laboratory technicians
- microbiologists
- physicians

hospitals. Genetic counselors who work in physician's private practices are paid only slightly less than those who work in private hospitals.

Benefits for genetic counselors depend on the employer. They might include paid vacation, sick days, personal days, health and dental insurance, and retirement savings plans.

WHAT IS THE JOB OUTLOOK?

This field is expected to grow much faster than average for many years to come. Scientific developments in understanding adult genetic disorders and in reproductive technologies have created new opportunities for treatment and testing. The data produced by the Human Genome Project (the mapping of human DNA) has created new ethical dilemmas as new genetic tests become available. This, in turn, will create an increased need for individuals who can help patients understand the options these developments present, as well as their associated risks. In addition, the new technology of pharmcogenetics, the study of how genetic differences affect patients' responses to medications, has created new opportunities for genetic counselors. Counselors are already involved in and will become more involved in setting up testing protocols, marketing, and business administration in this fast-growing specialty.

Health Advocates

SUMMARY

Definition
Due to the complex nature of today's insurance and health industries, patients turn to health advocates for help. Health advocates work on behalf of patients on issues ranging from insurance coverage to hospital intervention. Advocates are employed by hospitals and nonprofit groups, or work as independent contractors.

Alternative Job Titles
Consumer health advocates
Patient advocates
Patient relations managers
Patient representatives

Salary Range
$30,000 to $45,000 to $60,000

Educational Requirements
Bachelor's degree

Certification or Licensing
Voluntary

Outlook
Faster than the average

High School Subjects
Business
English (writing/literature)
Health
Mathematics
Speech

Personal Interests
Figuring out how things
    work
Fixing things
Helping people: emotionally
Helping people: physical
    health/medicine
Writing

"My personal history led me to a career in health care as I lost both of my parents to cancer before I was 18 years old," says Tammy Miller, a patient relations manager in Evansville, Indiana. "This experience formed a deep need in me to help patients and families face some of the most emotionally and physically difficult times of their lives. Patient advocates have opportunities every day to make a difference in the lives of the people that we serve."

WHAT DOES A HEALTH ADVOCATE DO?

Today's health care system has become very complex, and many patients often have difficulties navigating the maze of insurance plans and their limitations. *Health advocates*, using their health care and medical expertise, work on behalf of patients and their interests. Primarily, there are three types of health care advocates. Those who are employed by large companies such as hospitals, insurance companies, large physician groups, and other health organizations are often called *patient representatives,* or *consumer health advocates.* The second category of health advocates works primarily for nonprofit organizations that deal with a wide variety of medical and insurance concerns, or they might work for a group that targets a particular illness or disease, such as cancer or lupus. The third group of health advocates works for private advocacy firms.

Many hospitals have seen the need and benefits of having a team devoted to resolving complaints of patients and their families and watching out for the interests of the patients as well as of the hospital. Patient representatives receive complaints from the patient or the family and work towards a resolution to the problem. The problem may range from issues between two patients sharing a room, to miscommunication between the patient and medical staff, to misplaced personal items. If a patient feels mistreated by a hospital staff member, for example, the patient representative must hear both sides of the case, determine if the claim is valid or a misunderstanding, and hopefully work out a peaceful and satisfactory resolution.

Patient representatives also document patients' concerns and experience with the hospital and its staff. Complaints and the method of resolution are recorded to help in future cases. Measuring and recording patient satisfaction are important because the hospital uses this infor-

mation in finding areas to improve. Another important role of representatives is to interpret medical procedures or unfamiliar medical terms and to answer patients' questions in regards to hospital procedures or health insurance concerns. They also educate patients, as well as the hospital staff, about the patients' rights, advance directives, and issues of bioethics. Sometimes they handle special religious or dietary needs of the patient or personal requests, such as celebrating a birthday.

While patient representatives work for the patients' well-being as well as their employer's best interests, health advocates employed by nonprofits act as the patient's champion against insurance companies, employers, and creditors. Many times patients are denied much-needed medical treatments because insurance companies consider them to be experimental. Certain drugs might be denied because of the way they are taken. Health advocates provide assistance in getting these issues resolved. They help identify the type of health insurance and the depth of coverage the patient has, and organize paperwork and referrals from physicians and hospitals. Sometimes patients also need help composing letters to insurance companies explaining their situation. Health advocates also make phone calls to physicians and insurance companies on behalf of the patient.

Patients sometimes encounter job discrimination because of an existing illness or extended medical leaves, and this is another area in which health advocates

Lingo to Learn

advance directive A written communication to your family and health care providers stating your wishes about treatment if you are dying or no longer able to make health care decisions.

claim A request by an individual (or his or her health care provider) to an insurance company to pay for services of a health care provider.

denial of a claim Refusal by an insurance company to pay a claim submitted to them by a health care provider on behalf of an insured individual.

durable power of attorney for health care A legal document that allows a trusted family member or friend to act as an individual's proxy in making health care decisions.

living will A type of advance directive in which you put into writing your wishes about medical treatment should you be unable to communicate at the end of life. State laws may vary on when the living will goes into effect, and may limit the treatments to which the living will applies.

Patient Self-Determination Act An act passed by Congress in 1991 that requires all health facilities that receive federal funds to inform patients of their rights to accept or refuse treatment and to prepare advance directives.

can help. Many nonprofit groups also have lawyers on staff who provide legal counsel. Also, with any serious illness, financial concerns are likely. Health advocates can offer suggestions on how to get the most from a patient's insurance coverage, negotiate with physicians and hos-

pitals to lower costs, and work with pharmaceutical companies in providing expensive medications at a lower cost.

Health advocates may choose to work independent of a hospital, group, or organization. Such advocates act as consultants and may have their own private practice or work for an advocacy firm. Their cases usually involve patients with a variety of issues and concerns. They usually charge a flat fee per case.

WHAT IS IT LIKE TO BE A HEALTH ADVOCATE?

Tammy Miller works as a patient relations manager in Evansville, Indiana. She has been a hospital employee for 20 years, and a patient advocate for 15 years. In her current position, she oversees the patient relations programs at two sister hospitals: Deaconess Hospital and Deaconess Gateway Hospital. "I can't imagine another job that could be this rewarding in so many ways," Tammy says. "I have freedom and flexibility along with responsibility and authority. My opinion is valued by patients, families, and staff. At the end of each day, I feel that I truly made a difference."

Tammy describes her life as a patient advocate as a "roller coaster ride. I have the most unstructured day of any health care worker that I know. We may plan our day," she says, "but the next phone call or person who walks into our office can change everything. I would consider my main duties to be helping patients and families; taking, investigating, and resolving patient complaints and grievances; following up on patient surveys; coordinating volunteer visitors (hospital volunteers who we train to visit our patients during their hospitalization); searching for lost patient items (such as dentures, eyeglasses, hearing aids, etc.); coordinating our service-recovery process (if there is a minor breakdown in service, we offer the patient a sincere apology and a small token such as a meal or gas coupon); and looking for ways to improve our services and the overall patient experience."

DO I HAVE WHAT IT TAKES TO BE A HEALTH ADVOCATE?

The most important quality to have in this field is an intense desire to help others. As a health advocate, your central goal is to put the interest and needs of patients first. Being a good and compassionate listener is also important because you have to identify the patients' problem or fears before you can help them. You must also be prepared to interact with a variety of people, many times from different social and economic backgrounds. It is also important to have good communication skills. You must be able to effectively convey the patients' needs to insurance and pharmaceutical companies, but also be able to explain situations to patients clearly.

You must be aggressive and assertive. If the insurance company says no to a much-needed treatment, advocates need to find ways around the situation. The answer "no" must never be a deterrent. In

To Be a Successful Health Advocate, You Should . . .

- want to help others, especially those who can't help themselves
- be able to interact with people from a variety of social and economic backgrounds
- be a good speaker
- be a good listener
- be strong willed and aggressive
- be organized

these situations, having a health background may help give you an air of authority.

HOW DO I BECOME A HEALTH ADVOCATE?
Education
High School

Classes such as writing or public speaking help in this field. Health advocates spend a majority of their time talking with patients and employees of big organizations like major insurance companies. It's important to know how to express your message in a clear and concise manner. You may want to study biology or other health-related classes to get an understanding of the medical field. Although a medical background is not an absolute prerequisite, it is helpful to be familiar with common medical terms, diagnoses, and treatments.

Postsecondary Training

There are no nationally recognized education standards for health advocates. Most advocates have bachelor's degrees and experience in human services, communications, supervision, management, or conflict negotiation. Experience in health care is also important, including familiarity with medical terminology. Some advocates have degrees in social work or psychology and some are registered nurses. A few universities offer undergraduate courses in patient representation and a few, such as Sarah Lawrence College (http://www.slc.edu/home.php) in New York, have master's programs in health advocacy.

In addition to formal training, Tammy stresses the importance of lifelong learning. "A patient advocate is a lifelong learner because the health care environment is constantly changing," she says, "and we navigate the entire system and help families to navigate it as well. In addition, a patient advocate must stay current with the Centers for Medicare and Medicaid Services, the Joint Commission on Accreditation of Healthcare Organizations, and our state laws. Although most patient advocates have a bachelor's degree, we also keep up-to-date by being members of our state and national organizations as well as networking." [Tammy is on the board of directors of the Indiana Society for Healthcare Consumer Advocacy, served on the national Society for Healthcare Consumer Advocacy's (SHCA) board of directors,

The Patient Care Partnership

The American Hospital Association created this resource to ensure a safe and comfortable hospital stay and the best medical treatment possible. It is used as a guide for quality patient treatment at many hospitals and organizations. Highlights of *The Patient Care Partnership* include:

You, as the patient, have the right to considerate and respectful care.

You have the right to care in a clean and safe environment.

You have the right to know your diagnosis, treatment, and prognosis. You also have the right to know the identity of those treating you.

You have the right to advance directives—living will, power of attorney, and health care proxy.

You have the right to privacy, including medical records, test results, and examinations.

You have the right to refuse treatment, as well as the right to be informed of alternative care options.

To read the complete *Patient Care Partnership,* visit the association's Web site, http://www.aha.org/aha/ptcommunication/partnership/index.html.

and served as the program chair for the SHCA's national conference schedule in 2006.] "Patient advocates share freely information to help improve other hospitals' service to the customers; we are a true example of servant leadership."

Certification or Licensing

There is no one nationally recognized certification program offered for this field. Continuing education classes are offered throughout the year for those already in the field; for example, advocates might attend seminars covering topics such as hospital ethics, changes in Medicare or Medicaid, and computer training.

Internships and Volunteerships

If you want a career in health advocacy, but are undecided which route to take, consider an internship. Families USA (http://www.familiesusa.org), for example, offers several paid internships to college students, graduate students, and recent graduates. Prerequisites include a strong academic background and an interest in public education, advocacy, and media relations. Interns work on projects such as monitoring government policy changes on Medicare and Medicaid and preparing educational information on health and welfare issues for community leaders and the public.

If you want to gain work experience while in high school, you may find volunteer opportunities at your local nursing home or hospital. Time spent at a nursing home, for example, can prepare you to interact with the elderly. You may be asked to run errands or perform small tasks such as writing letters for those without relatives living nearby.

Many nonprofit advocacy groups welcome volunteers to do a variety of tasks. You may be assigned to collate informational flyers or participate in a fund-raiser

instead of heading an actual grievance case; however, the work experience and industry contacts are invaluable.

WHO WILL HIRE ME?

Your future employment depends on the field of advocacy you wish to pursue. Do you want a regular Monday-through-Friday schedule, a hospital environment, and a customer-service work setting? If so, then your main employers will be hospitals, specialty practices, and managed-care organizations. Nonprofit organizations, such as foundations dealing with a particular illness like cancer or a special group such as the elderly, hire advocates to handle patients' treatment needs or financial difficulties.

WHERE CAN I GO FROM HERE?

Health advocates who work as members of a staff in a hospital can advance to department manager or other administrative positions. Some health advocates may find jobs in hospices or in AIDS programs. With solid work experience and expertise in a particular field, you may be a candidate for advocacy work on a national level. High-profile advocates travel extensively, giving speeches or seminars or familiarizing members of Congress on a particular cause.

In the next five years, Tammy would like to become the president of the Society for Healthcare Consumer Advocacy. "I would like to co-author a book, for sale nationally, that explains the importance of our role in the health care experience. A goal would also be to help write grants to enable more patient advocates to increase their knowledge base through education. Within the next 10 years, I would like to teach a college-level course in the health care curriculum focused on improving the patient/family experience."

WHAT ARE THE SALARY RANGES?

Advocates working for hospitals, insurance companies, or large group practices earn between $40,000 and $60,000 a year. Those employed in the private sector also enjoy benefits such as paid vacation and sick time, some overtime pay, health insurance, and retirement plans. Since most nonprofit groups are without the financial means of private corporations, most advocates working for nonprofits tend to earn much less.

Independent health advocates have opportunities that employed advocates do not—working solely for the benefit of the patient, setting their own hours, and working from home. Independents, however, do not have the stability of job security or a regular monthly salary. Self-employed health advocates usually work for consultant fees that range from $75 to $150 per case. After analyzing insurance statements and identifying any savings for the patient, that amount is split evenly between the patient and the advocate. Though many self-employed advocates enjoy a good salary, it is certainly unpredictable; independents may have many clients and referrals one year

It's Good to Be Organized

Advocates encourage patients to be organized. It's important to keep copies of all paperwork connected with health care, including medical records, test results, physician referrals, documentation, and correspondence from hospitals and insurance companies. They suggest organizing paperwork according to subject matter and keeping all information in one binder. Having all information on hand makes the advocate's job and the patient's case easier to complete.

and a slow year with little earnings the next.

WHAT IS THE JOB OUTLOOK?

The U.S. Department of Labor expects that as many as 3.6 million jobs will be created in health care services through 2014, listing it as one the fastest growing major industry groups. Although health advocacy is only a small part of this industry, it would be safe to assume that employment of health advocates will also grow. As insurance, hospital, and medical services become more advanced and complex, patients' need for advocates will increase as well.

As insurance issues become more complicated, people will turn to experts to interpret the legalese and show results. Health advocates can provide this guidance and get attention paid to their patients' cases, especially from big bureaucracies like Medicare and other insurance giants. As the number of health advocates grows, there will be more regulations, and perhaps a national standard of certification and training will develop to better establish the field of health advocacy.

Health Care Managers

SUMMARY

Definition
Health care managers run hospitals and other health care organizations that provide patient care.

Alternative Job Titles
Department managers
Hospital administrators
Nursing home administrators

Salary Range
$42,300 to $68,320 to $117,730+

Educational Requirements
Bachelor's degree;
    master's degree strongly recommended

Certification or Licensing
Voluntary (certification)
Required for certain positions (licensing)

Outlook
Faster than the average

High School Subjects
Business

English (writing/literature)
Mathematics

Personal Interests
Business management
Economics
Helping people: physical health/medicine

Unfortunately, there is no shortage of injury and illness in the world. "The challenge," says Samuel Odle, a health care administrator in Indianapolis, Indiana, "is that people want high-quality health care, but they either want to pay less for it [payors] or they lack the resources to pay for the care they need [uninsured citizens]. Staying true to your mission of providing the highest quality patient care to everyone, regardless of their ability to pay, is the greatest challenge. But it's also the energizing part of the job that causes you to keep thinking of creative ways to be successful from a business standpoint so you can continue to serve. In the end, that's what health care is about—serving our fellow citizens, at what is usually their most vulnerable time in life. This is the challenge and the reward of a career in health care."

WHAT DOES A HEALTH CARE MANAGER DO?

Health care managers oversee health care facilities or individual departments within them. Management positions range from middle-management department heads to senior-level managers. Health care managers are accountable for the financial side of the business. Similar to other business managers, health care managers plan, organize, supervise, budget, and direct staff. They develop and implement programs and services, manage their employees and physical facilities, identify and solve problems, and develop budgets. Health care managers are responsible for establishing fees and billing procedures, planning space needs, purchasing supplies and equipment, and providing mail, phone, computer, laundry, and other services needed by patients and staff. Working with other medical staff and department heads, they may also develop and implement training programs for staff members.

To accomplish their many duties, health care managers meet regularly with staff members and colleagues to discuss pressing issues, expectations, and recent accomplishments. They may also be actively involved in the community, attending meetings or making speeches to community groups and professional organizations. Managers may be required to travel to their organization's regional facilities or to out-of-town meetings.

Health care organizations are varied, ranging from single hospitals to multi-hospital systems, nursing homes, clinics, hospices, health maintenance organizations, medical group practices, mental health centers, ambulatory care facilities, and rehabilitation centers. In small facilities, health care managers usually handle all the management responsibilities, taking a more direct role in daily operations. In large facilities, the *chief executive officer* (CEO) in charge of managing the entire organization delegates duties to other administrators; for example, a CEO may assign personnel matters to the facility's human resources manager.

Health care managers may be *generalists* (in charge of an entire facility) or *specialists* (in charge of specific clinical departments or services). Examples of areas within health care facilities that have specialized managers include clinical areas such as surgery, nursing, physical therapy, and psychiatry, and administrative areas such as finance, security, maintenance, and housekeeping.

Generalists have broader managerial responsibilities and, as a result, require a more comprehensive background. On the other hand, specialists must be trained and educated in the area they manage. Nursing administrators, for example, generally have worked as staff nurses before advancing into management. Similarly, most medical records administrators hold a bachelor's degree in medical records administration.

Hospital administrators are generalists who work with the institution's governing board to develop long-range plans and policy. Administrators are accountable for the success of business plans, such as proposals to expand health care services or implement a fund-raising campaign. Administrators set the overall direction of the organization. They deal with government regulation, reimbursement, and community issues.

Department managers are responsible for staff, budgets, programs, and policies for their specific area. They may coordinate activities with other managers.

Group medical practice managers work closely with the physician owners. *Office managers* usually handle business matters for small group practices, while physicians make policy decisions. Large medical group practices, however, often hire a full-time health care administrator to manage the business operation and delegate responsibilities to assistants.

Health maintenance organization (HMO) managers have responsibilities similar to managers in large group medical practices but may have larger staffs. They also may put more emphasis on preventive care.

The health care field has undergone tremendous changes over the past several years. These changes include the merging and restructuring of health care institutions. The number of stand-alone hospitals has decreased, while the number of hospital systems continues to grow. Health care managers are (and will continue to be) involved in the restructuring of health care organizations; they must have concern for both fiscal management as well as patient care.

Though similar in nature to other administrative or management positions, health care managers have the rare opportunity to help improve the health of the communities in which they serve. They accomplish this by researching the demographics of the communities, determining their needs, providing relevant services, and promoting these services in the community.

WHAT IS IT LIKE TO BE A HEALTH CARE MANAGER?

Samuel Odle has worked in the health care industry for 39 years. "I came to the hospital looking for a job," he recalls. "I found an environment that was compatible with my desire to work with people and be helpful. After a few weeks, I knew the hospital environment was a match for me."

Samuel's first job in health care was as an X-ray technician. He then completed a degree in allied health education. His first significant management position was as a director of a department of radiology. "During that time," he says, "I completed a master's in health care administration and have had various administrative-level positions in my career." Samuel currently serves as executive vice president for Clarian Health and President and CEO of Methodist and Indiana University Hospitals in Indianapolis, Indiana.

Samuel's basic responsibilities are to provide operational and strategic direc-

Advancement Possibilities

- *Department managers* are responsible for a specific area that provides patient care or support services.

- *Administrators* are responsible for the overall direction of a hospital or other health care facility.

- *Chief executive officers* are in charge of the operation of a large health care facility or system.

tion for two adult hospitals and strategic direction for an eight-hospital system. "I usually arrive early in the morning at my office, check e-mails, and send out whatever communications I need to start the day," he explains. "I then spend the day in meetings, reviewing operational performance, discussing problems, and help to develop solutions for them. I spend a great deal of time working with medical staff to help balance our tripartite mission of education, research, and clinical care. Many of the meetings I participate in have to do with the allocation of resources (i.e., money). We are always evaluating whether we are getting the right return on our investment. Are we investing in the right things—capital and people? What do we need to plan on investing in the future?"

Another aspect of Samuel's job is interacting with external organizations. "Sometimes these are health care organizations that you are coordinating activities with," he explains. "We also have a number of contacts with governmental and regulatory organizations to be sure we stay in compliance."

Samuel also serves on several standing committees, such as Patient Quality and Risk Management. "Our core product is clinical care. Participating in these meetings allows me to stay close to the end results of our actions," he says. "I also work with the board of directors and the CEO and the CFO of the health system to do strategic planning to ensure we are taking a system view. I also review performance metrics to ensure the final outcome of our work, the health status of our community, is improving."

Alyson Pitman Giles began her career in health care as an occupational therapist in 1977, and moved into health care management in rehabilitation shortly thereafter. She is currently the president and CEO of CMC Healthcare System and Catholic Medical Center in Manchester, New Hampshire. "The joy of my work life as president and CEO of Catholic Medical Center," she says, "is that every day is different. Literally, there is no 'typical day.' When you are an occupational therapist, your productivity is measured by your direct patient care contact. As a CEO, productivity is measured by the overall strategy and success of the organization."

Alyson spends approximately 25 percent of her time in meetings with board members. "We have a full board meeting once a month," she says, "and numerous committee meetings in finance, strategic planning, research, credentialing, quality, etc. throughout the month. She spends another 25 percent of her time with the medical staff, where she deals with issues such as quality, credentialing, recruitment, and problem solving. "I work closely with not only medical staff leaders, but physicians from all different specialties to help them to have the best possible experience working at my hospital," she says. "Another 25 percent of my time is spent managing and supervising the leadership team of Catholic Medical Center. We have more than 1,700 employees and 400 physicians in the organization. I have a senior management team of eight individuals and approximately eight direct reports. My job is to oversee their work and to cultivate the talent within the organization. I also meet directly with employees and managers in a number of venues.

Alyson spends the remaining 25 percent of her day working on the strategy and the future of the organization, and in outreach to community organizations. "I serve on many boards and, essentially, serve as a link between the hospital and the greater community," she explains. "Not only can I provide expertise and time to community organizations, but I am the constant face of Catholic Medical Center within the state of New Hampshire."

DO I HAVE WHAT IT TAKES TO BE A HEALTH CARE MANAGER?

"The personal and professional qualities that health care leaders need," according to Alyson Pitman Giles, "are the ability to communicate with people and to recognize and cultivate talent. Successful leaders need to be able to see an organization from one hundred thousand feet, as well as from the ground level. Health care leaders must be willing to be ongoing learners to continue to evolve and change as the environment changes around them. I try to meet all new employees attending the organization's orientation program and all new managers. I propose that they always 'maintain their humility, their gratitude, and keep in mind that no matter what they hear, there is always another side to every story.' This advice is fundamental, but critical to success and job satisfaction."

Lingo to Learn

ambulatory care A facility that treats patients on an outpatient basis.

HMO (health maintenance organization) A prepaid managed care plan where members pay a fixed amount of money in exchange for most of their medical needs.

hospice A facility that provides health care, especially pain control and emotional support, to terminally ill patients and their families.

managed care A system for organizing many health care providers within a single organization to control health care costs.

nursing home A facility that provides living quarters and care for persons unable to look after themselves, such as the elderly or chronically ill.

PPO (preferred provider organization) A managed care medical plan that contracts with doctors, hospitals, and other providers to obtain discounts for care. Providers agree on a predetermined list of fees for all services.

rehabilitation center A facility that uses therapy, education, and emotional support to help patients regain health to lead useful lives.

Health care managers must be able to work effectively with people at all levels in the organization—governing board members, medical staff, senior management, other managers, subordinates—as well as patients and their families, community leaders, and vendors. Their many responsibilities require tact and good judgment.

Health care managers require administrative skills such as the ability to train, delegate, evaluate, and negotiate with staff. In addition, they must be able to coordinate a variety of functions concurrently.

Leadership skills are also necessary to inspire and motivate others. Health care managers have to weather some disappointments (failures in the system or being let down by staff members or colleagues) occasionally.

Managers must also have analytical skills to be able to understand and solve problems quickly. However, at other times, they must show patience and thoroughness when a decision needs more thought and careful research. To solve many of their problems, health care managers must understand financial management, information systems, human resources, public relations, marketing, and organizational behavior.

Finally, they must also be interested in health care and in management.

HOW DO I BECOME A HEALTH CARE MANAGER?
Education
Samuel Odle has a bachelor's degree in allied health education and a master's degree in health care administration. "My educational training has helped me since a great deal of management is teaching and counseling," he says. "My health administration degree helps me understand the bigger picture, but most of my skills have been developed by on-the-job training. Health care is a rapidly chang-

ing business and you must continue your education throughout your career."

When Alyson Pitman Giles entered the field of health care, she did so somewhat by accident. "In my freshman year in college," she recalls, "I was closed out of the biology 101 class and was forced into an anatomy and physiology course. It was very clear to me that I needed to be involved in direct patient care in health care. I transferred as a junior into occupational therapy and soon moved into rehabilitation management. I received mostly on-the-job training until I went into a graduate program in human service administration, which I completed in 1988."

High School
Students considering a career in health care management should take science, math, and business courses. Since both oral and written communication skills are required, English and speech classes are recommended. Samuel advises students interested in health care management to get a part-time job in a hospital. "Find out if the environment is the right place for you," he says. "If it is, keep working, get your formal education, and look for a job that allows you to express yourself. If you find something within health care that you like to do, you will be good at it, and the income and benefits will take care of themselves."

Postsecondary Training
Health care managers must hold a minimum of a bachelor's degree for entry-level positions in smaller facilities or

departments. Entry-level health care managers move into higher positions through work experience or after obtaining additional education.

Most senior management positions require a master's degree in health services administration, medical administration, or public health, although some managers are entering the field with graduate degrees in medicine, business, public administration, and other fields.

To earn a master's degree, students complete course work in areas such as hospital organization and management, marketing, human resources, accounting, strategic planning, and health information systems. In addition, most programs require that students complete an internship or residency, and possibly write a thesis.

Some programs allow students to specialize in a particular type of organization, such as hospitals, nursing homes, mental health facilities, health maintenance organizations, or ambulatory care facilities. Other programs provide a generalist approach to health care administration.

Health care managers who want to teach, consult, or conduct research may be required to hold a Ph.D.

According to the Association of University Programs in Health Administration, there are approximately 150 undergraduate and graduate programs in health care administration in North America.

In addition to formal education, health care managers must continue to learn throughout their careers. "Health care leaders have to be committed to lifelong learning," Samuel advises. "Your professional association is the best way for you to get the additional learning and to benchmark yourself against your peers in the field. It's also a good opportunity for networking and mentoring, allowing you to improve your leadership skills after you have received your formal education."

Alyson agrees that continuing education and professional development is key to success in this career. "I have progressed from a member to a diplomate and on to become a fellow of the American College of Healthcare Executives (ACHE)," she says. "ACHE has provided a foundation of colleagues and ongoing education to prepare me for my career."

Certification or Licensing

Managers working as nursing home administrators are required to be licensed by the state in which they practice. Requirements vary depending on the state, but generally, nursing home managers must obtain a bachelor's degree from an accredited college or university, complete a state-approved training program, and pass a licensing examination. They must also complete continuing education courses and renew their license yearly or every two years.

State licensing is not required for other health care managers. Certification, offered by the American College of Health Care Administrators and the American College of Healthcare Executives, is voluntary. Managers may choose to obtain certification to improve their professional credibility and opportunities for advancement.

Interview

Brigadier General David Rubenstein is the Assistant Surgeon General for Force Sustainment, U.S. Army at Headquarters, U.S. Army Medical Command, Fort Sam Houston, in San Antonio, Texas. He has served in the army since May 1977, and has been the Assistant Surgeon General since July 2005. His specialty before becoming a general officer was as a health care administrator.

Q. Why did you decide to enter this career?

A. I entered the army because I was offered an ROTC scholarship to fund my undergraduate degree. I chose the Medical Service Corps in order to help soldiers and their families to have the ability to set the environment for clinicians to provide high quality health care, to serve the country, and to learn a skill that would be transferable to a career after the army.

Q. Tell us about a day in your work life.

A. I have a portfolio that is global in nature and applies to both the Army Medical Department's (AMEDD) mission at home and on the battlefield. I'm responsible for information management, information technology, medical logistics, installation and facility management, and health care contracting in support of the Army Medical Department's mission of caring for more than three million beneficiaries. In my present position, I give broad guidance and provide coaching to senior health care executives who are directly responsible for each of the portfolio areas. A typical day starts with a physical fitness regime before attending a video-tele-conference among AMEDD leaders in San Antonio, Texas, and Washington, D.C. The remaining hours of the day are spent in meetings and attending to paperwork and e-mail. My additional duty is to represent the army's surgeon general and the AMEDD at meetings, conferences, and events around the country

Q. How did you train for this career?

A. I graduated from Texas A&M University with a bachelor's degree in community health education. The army then provided appropriate training in time for each new assignment during my 29-year career. I also earned a master's degree in health administration from Baylor University to serve as the foundation for my career as a health care administrator. I've also earned a master's degree in military art and science with a history concentration.

Q. Where do you see yourself professionally in the next decade?

A. I will have retired from the army in the next 10 years and will be working in a civilian health care setting, either in a hospital or other patient care organization, or in the corporate headquarters of a health care system.

Q. What advice would you give to high school students who are interested in careers in health care management?

A. Health care management is a wonderful way to ensure that your community has the very best health care available. Health care executives set the

(continued on next page)

(continued from previous page)

framework to ensure that quality health care is available for a community.

Q. What advice would you give to students who are interested in pursuing careers in the military?

A. The military is an ideal way to gain the knowledge, skills, and experiences that health care organizations are looking for in their seasoned senior executives. The military provides many rich opportunities to gain critical interpersonal, leadership, and hands-on management skills early in a career. These experiences are invaluable and come much earlier in a military career then they do in a civilian health care management career.

Internships and Volunteerships

During supervised internships or residencies, students can apply the theories and principles they learned in class to the type of health care setting in which they want to work. The administrators with whom the students work closely serve as their mentors. Some programs may also include a fellowship, which involves additional supervised work.

Alyson advises high school students to "volunteer in hospitals and get to see some of the different areas and 'walk in the shoes' of some of the different health care professions. Not only would volunteer work supplement their portfolio, but they can develop relationships that could ultimately lead to jobs."

Related Jobs

- city managers
- college administrators
- financial institution officers and managers
- hotel and motel managers
- management analysts and consultants
- nurse managers
- office administrators
- property and real estate managers
- restaurant and food service managers
- retail business owners
- retail managers

WHO WILL HIRE ME?

Approximately 248,000 health care managers are employed in the United States. Health care managers work in a variety of settings. Besides hospitals and hospital systems, positions can be found in ambulatory care facilities, hospices, nursing homes, health maintenance organizations, medical group practices, mental health organizations, universities, public health departments, consulting firms, and health care associations. In addition, health care managers work in home health agencies, dentists' offices, medical and dental laboratories, and offices of allied health professionals.

Most universities have career services offices that offer their students and graduates information about career opportunities as well as specific job openings.

Many people learn about job openings by joining professional membership organizations. Membership allows managers to network with other members and find out about conferences, continuing education, and other professional activities. The American College of Healthcare Executives (ACHE) offers a student associate membership with a reduced membership fee. These student chapters invite guest speakers, elect officers, and undertake community service and fundraising projects.

Job openings can also be found in the classified advertising sections of newspapers in major cities. In addition, executive search firms that recruit for the health care field may help in locating management positions. In many cases, the employer pays any applicable fees to the recruiter.

WHERE CAN I GO FROM HERE?

Advancement in health care management usually depends on a combination of a person's education and experience and the organization's size and complexity. A health care manager's first job may be an entry-level to mid-level management position in a specialized area such as patient care services, medical staff relations, or finance. Once they have experience, health care managers can move into positions with higher levels of responsibility, such as chief executive officer, administrator, assistant administrator, vice president, or department manager. Those with master's degrees have better opportunities for advancing into higher-level positions. Knowledge of and experience in finance, budgeting, information systems, strategic planning, patient care, and staff management are valuable.

Keys to advancement are keeping informed of the changes in the field and staying flexible to take advantage of opportunities when they appear. One way to advance your career is to take on greater responsibility.

Samuel Odle says that he is committed to his current health system and the community it serves. "I anticipate being here for the next 10 years. I anticipate we will be a larger health system, so there will be new and bigger challenges for me."

"I see myself continuing in a president and CEO position for at least the next five years in my current organization," Alyson Pitman Giles predicts. "At that time, I will either move into a foundation role or will consider doing some interim CEO positions to help organizations prepare for new leadership."

WHAT ARE THE SALARY RANGES?

Salaries of health services executives depend on the type of facility, geographic location, the size of the administrative staff, the budget, and the policy of the governing board. The U.S. Department of Labor reports that the median annual earnings of medical and health services managers were $68,320 in 2004. Salaries ranged from less than $42,300 to more than $117,730. Health care managers who worked in hospitals had mean annual earnings of $78,480 and those who worked in nursing and personal care facilities earned $65,660.

Some administrators receive free meals, housing, and laundry service, depending on the facility in which they are employed. They usually receive paid vacations and holidays, sick leave, hospitalization and insurance benefits, and pension programs. The executive benefits package nowadays often includes management incentive bonuses based on job

To Be a Successful Health Care Manager, You Should . . .

- have excellent communication skills

- a good eye for talent

- have excellent leadership and management skills

- have strong analytical skills

- have good knowledge of mathematics and business management

- be committed to providing quality, cost-effective health care to those you serve

performance ranging from $25,000 to $225,000.

WHAT IS THE JOB OUTLOOK?

"People who are looking for a career that is as much like a ministry as it is a job will find health care to be exciting, challenging, and rewarding," says Samuel Odle. "If you are the type of person who wants to make a difference in the lives of individuals and in the world, health care is the place to be." The health care field today is dynamic and growing, offering a wide range of opportunities and challenges. Employment for health care managers is expected to grow faster than the average for all occupations, according to the U.S. Department of Labor. The health care industry is expanding because of the growing aging population, advances in medical technology, increasing emphasis on disease prevention, and growing pressures from business, government, insurance companies, and patients to hold down health care costs. "I think the health care field is a wide-open arena that should be considered by all students in high school," says Alyson Pitman Giles. "There are terrific jobs in radiology, nursing, pharmacy, and the therapies. In addition, there are outstanding opportunities for those with an MBA or a MHA to move into health care management."

Job opportunities are available at a variety of organizational levels, from chief executive officer to department head. Health care managers with strong business and management skills will find the best job opportunities. Those with graduate degrees will also have an edge.

Competition for top jobs is intense, but because of the expansion and diversification of health care services, employment will grow in nontraditional areas that provide patient care. The best opportunities for health care managers will be in general medical and surgical hospitals and offices of health practitioners. In addition, health maintenance organizations are being marketed to elderly citizens to supplement or replace Medicare programs. Growth in this market will increase the need for qualified health care managers. In addition, job prospects are increasing in ambulatory care as patients receive more health care services on an outpatient basis. Finally, the long-term care segment of the industry is expanding to meet the needs of the rapidly growing elderly population. Patients are demanding (and receiving) more specialized high-quality services geared to their individual needs. This demand has lead to the growth of patient care services specifically designed for the elderly, women, and children.

Medical and Science Writers and Editors

SUMMARY

Definition
Medical and science writers research and interpret technical, scientific, and medical information and then write about it in such a way as to make it accessible to the appropriate audience—the general public or professionals in the field. Medical and science editors perform a wide range of functions, but their primary responsibility is to ensure that text provided by writers is suitable in content, format, and style for the intended audiences. Readers are the first priority of writers and editors.

Alternative Job Titles
None

Salary Range
$23,700 to $57,800 to $87,660+

Educational Requirements
Bachelor's degree

Certification or Licensing
Voluntary

Outlook
About as fast as the average

High School Subjects
English (writing/literature)
Health
Journalism
Science

Personal Interests
Current events
Helping people: physical health/medicine
Science
Writing

One of James Cozzarin's most memorable experiences as a medical editor was assisting a pharmaceutical company prepare for its presentation at a Food and Drug Administration (FDA) advisory committee meeting (ACM). (An ACM is where the FDA hears arguments for and against granting approval for a new drug to be sold to the public).

"The product was a new drug designed to treat a disease for which there was previously no treatment," James recalls. "To make a long story short, we were success-

ful in our efforts, and the drug was approved for sale. What did this mean to the public? It meant that on the day before the ACM, if you had this disease, you were likely to die from it. On the day after the drug was approved, if you had this disease, you could be treated."

"What did this mean to me? It meant everything! To play even a small part in helping to bring a new drug to the public, to help put a therapy in the hands of patients for whom there was no available treatment, was nothing short of miraculous! Times like these, albeit rare, remind me of the importance of our work and of the dramatic effect we can have on a large number of people. It's part of what attracted me to this career in the beginning, and it's a large part of why I have continued to find my work both professionally and personally rewarding for more than a decade."

WHAT DOES A MEDICAL/SCIENCE WRITER OR EDITOR DO?

As our world becomes more complex and people seek even more information, professional writers and editors have become increasingly important. And, as medicine and science take giant steps forward and discoveries are being made every day that affect our lives, skilled *medical and science writers and editors* are needed to document these changes and disseminate the information to the general public and more specialized audiences. Because the medical and scientific subject areas may sometimes overlap, writers often find that they do science writing as well as medical writing. A medical writer, for instance, may write about a scientific study that has an impact on the medical field.

According to Jeanie Davis, former president of the Southeast Chapter of the American Medical Writers Association (AMWA), "Medical writing can take several different avenues. You may be a consumer medical writer, write technical medical research, or write about health care issues. Some choose to be medical editors and edit reports written by researchers. Sometimes this medical research must be translated into reports and news releases that the public can understand. Today, many writers write for the Web." She adds, "It is a very dynamic profession, always changing."

Some medical and science writers specialize in their subject matter. A medical writer may write only about heart disease and earn a reputation as one of the best writers in that particular area. Science writers may limit their writing or research to environmental science subjects, or they may be even more specific and focus only on air pollution issues.

Depending on their employment status, medical and science writers may be given a specific writing assignment by their editor or client. An experienced writer with contacts may pitch, or suggest, a story idea to a medical or science magazine, or a newspaper with a section devoted to medicine or science. In order to pitch a story idea, writers first have to develop a relevant, interesting topic based on their ongoing research into advancements in science and medicine. One way to stay on top of what's happening in medicine or science is to read industry magazines. Many medical and science writers read *Science, Nature,* the *Journal of the American Medical Association, The New England Journal of Medicine, Discover,* and *New Scientist.*

Writers always need good background information regarding a subject before they can write about it. To gain a thorough understanding of the subject matter, medical and science writers may spend hours doing research on the Internet or in corporate, university, or public libraries. Medical and science conferences also offer a wealth of information, so writers frequently attend them in search of topic ideas or data. They often supplement this research by conducting interviews with professionals such as doctors, pharmacists, scientists, engineers, managers, and other experts.

It's also important to present the information so it can be understood. This requires knowing the audience, whether it is the general public or professionals in medicine or science. Once medical and science writers have collected background material, they organize everything into a logical order. Medical and science writers who write for the general public translate high-tech information into articles and reports that are accurate and easily understood.

Lingo to Learn

byline Line appearing in an article or story giving the name of the writer.

clip Published work sample usually clipped from a publication.

pitch To suggest a story idea to a publication hoping that it will be accepted and then printed.

portfolio Collection of clips (news stories, magazine articles, or other pieces written) that serve as work samples for a person seeking employment.

trade journal Periodical having content geared toward members of a particular industry.

Some medical and science writers must be skilled in public relations. These writers report on advances made by their employers (for example, research facilities, government agencies, or high-tech companies) in such a way as to promote their work. Other writers try to remain unbiased in their reporting, illustrating to their readers both the pros and the cons of the medical or scientific achievements they're writing about so that readers can evaluate the merits of each particular achievement for themselves.

An article may be enhanced by the use of graphs, photos, or sidebars containing historical facts. Writers sometimes enlist the help of technical or medical illustrators or engineers to add a visual dimension to their work. If reporting on a new heart surgery procedure that will soon be available to the public, writers may need to discuss how that surgery is performed and which areas of the heart are affected. They may give a basic overview of how the healthy heart works, show a diseased heart in comparison, and report on how this surgery can help the patient. The public will also want to know how many people are affected by this disease, what the symptoms are, how many procedures have been done successfully, where they were performed, what the recovery time is, and if there are any complications. In addition, interviews with doctors and patients add a personal touch to the story.

Writers for broadcast media need to write short, precise articles that can be transmitted in a specific time allotment. They need to work quickly because news-related stories are often deadline oriented. Writing for the Web encompasses most journalistic guidelines including time constraints and sometimes space constraints.

Some writers choose to be freelance writers either on a full- or part-time basis or to supplement other jobs. Freelance medical and science writers are self-employed writers who work with small and large companies, health care organizations, research institutions, and publishing firms on a contract or hourly basis. They may specialize in writing about a specific medical or scientific subject for one or two clients, or they may write about a broad range of subjects for a number of different clients.

Medical and science editors work for many kinds of publishers, publications, and organizations. Editors' titles vary widely, not only from one area of publishing to another but also within each area. *Book editors* prepare written material for publication. In small publishing houses, the same editor may guide the material through all the stages of the publishing process. They may work with typesetters, printers, designers, advertising agencies, and other members of the publishing industry. In larger publishing houses, editors tend to be more specialized, being involved in only a part of the publishing process.

Acquisitions editors are the editors who find new writers and sign on new projects. They are responsible for finding new ideas for books that will sell well and for finding writers who can create the books.

Production editors are responsible for taking the manuscript written by an author and polishing the work into a finished book. They correct grammar, spelling, and style, and check all the facts. They make sure the book reads well and suggest changes to the author if it does not. The production editor may be responsible for getting the cover designed and the art put into a book. Because the work is so demanding, production editors usually work on only one or two books at a time.

Copy editors assist the production editor in polishing the author's writing. Copy editors review each page and make all the changes required to give the book a good writing style. *Line editors* review the text to make sure specific style rules are obeyed. They make sure the same spelling is used for words where more than one spelling is correct (for example, *grey* and *gray*).

The basic functions performed by *magazine* and *newspaper editors* are much like those performed by book editors, but a significant amount of the writing that appears in magazines and newspapers, or periodicals, is done by staff writers. Periodicals often use editors who specialize in specific areas, such as medical editors, who oversee the work of reporters who specialize in medical and science topics, and *department editors.* Department editors specialize in areas such as medicine, science, business, fashion, sports, and features, to name only a few. These departments are determined by the interests of the audience that the periodical intends to reach. Like book houses, periodicals use copy editors,

To Be a Successful Medical or Science Writer or Editor, You Should . . .

- enjoy learning, reading, and writing
- have an insatiable curiosity
- enjoy talking to people
- be able to deal with deadline pressure
- be persistent
- have strong interest in science and medicine
- have excellent organizational skills

researchers, and fact checkers, but at small periodicals, one or a few editors may be responsible for tasks that would be performed by many people at a larger publication.

WHAT IS IT LIKE TO BE A MEDICAL/SCIENCE WRITER OR EDITOR?

James Cozzarin is the manager of the editorial services team at ProEd Communications Inc., a health science communications firm in Beachwood, Ohio. He has worked at ProEd for more than 11 years. Before he became manager, he served in a variety of positions, including lead editor, senior medical editor, medical editor,

and copy editor. James also is the president-elect of the American Medical Writers Association. "I have long had a love of the English language," he says, "having written and edited prose and poetry in high school and college. I also have a love of science and medicine, and even spent two years in a nursing program in college before transferring to the college of education, where I received my degree. It was the combination of these two passions—English and medicine—that prompted me to enter this career."

James has a variety of duties as manager of the editorial services team at ProEd. "As manager of the team," he says, "I am responsible for everything the team does on a daily basis, as well as annual and quarterly planning, forecasting, personnel management, and inter-team communications. As a medical editor, I am also responsible for accurate and efficient editorial work, including research, fact checking, substantive editing, copy editing, style editing, proofreading, and quality control. As a senior member of the team, I am also involved in orientation and training of new employees, ongoing training and professional development of existing employees, and interviewing of candidates. I have also been called upon to support the medical writing staff by writing primary and review articles, as well as nonscientific pieces such as staff and faculty biographies, meeting collateral materials, evaluations, and post-tests."

Generally, writers and editors work in an office or research environment. Writers may travel in order to gather research information and conduct interviews. Certain employers may confine research to local libraries or the Internet. In addition, some employers require writers to conduct research interviews over the phone rather than in person.

Although the workweek usually runs 35 to 40 hours in a normal office setting, many writers and editors may have to work overtime to cover a story, interview people, meet deadlines, or disseminate information in a timely manner. The newspaper and broadcasting industries deliver the news 24 hours a day, seven days a week. Writers and editors often work nights and weekends to meet press deadlines or to cover a late-developing story.

DO I HAVE WHAT IT TAKES TO BE A MEDICAL/SCIENCE WRITER OR EDITOR?

Writers and editors should be able to express ideas clearly, have a broad general knowledge, be skilled in research techniques, and be computer literate. For some jobs—on a newspaper, for example, where the activity is hectic and deadlines short—the ability to concentrate and produce under pressure is essential.

You must be detail oriented to succeed as a writer or an editor. You must also be patient, since you may have to spend hours synthesizing information into the written word or turning a few pages of near-gibberish into powerful, elegant English. If you are the kind of person who can't sit still, you probably will not succeed in these careers. To be a good writer or editor, you must be a self-starter who is not afraid to make decisions. You must be good not only at identifying problems but also at solving them, so you must be creative.

It's not essential that you take every science or health course available in school, but you should at least have a solid grasp of and interest in basic science. Without an interest in medicine or science, a writer or editor may become bored or feel incapable of producing content that appeals to the target audience. You should be curious and take pleasure in learning new things since medicine and science are ever changing. Good writers who cover their subjects thoroughly have inquisitive minds and enjoy looking for additional information that might enhance their articles. Persistence comes in handy if data or people are hard to track down.

Freelancers should be resourceful in scouting out a range of publishers to whom they can submit article ideas. They should also be self-motivated. It is up to the freelance writer to keep track of deadlines and to garner enough assignments to make ends meet financially. An enjoyment of working alone is also vital. But medical and science writers and editors considering a freelance career should be aware that it's a lot of hard work and can become very isolating no matter how much a person likes to be alone.

HOW DO I BECOME A MEDICAL/SCIENCE WRITER OR EDITOR?
Education

There are many paths that lead to a career as a medical/science writer or editor. Some people develop an early interest in writing or editing and later discover an interest in medicine or science, while for others the reverse might be true. And still others may simultaneously become interested in writing or editing and in medicine or science. Often those who become medical/science writers and editors start out working in another field entirely. That was the case for James, who earned a bachelor of science in education, with a major in English and a minor in general science, from Kent State University in Kent, Ohio. "I was fortunate to find a teaching job immediately upon graduation," he recalls, "and for the next five years I taught junior high and high school English. During this time, I became interested in a career in publishing, where I could further sharpen my English skills." James accepted a position with Banks-Baldwin Law Publishing in Cleveland, Ohio, where he worked and trained as an editor. "One of my favorite projects while there was taking the lead on the *Ohio Nursing Law* practice book," he says. "My love of science and medicine never waned, and I eventually pursued and obtained a position with ProEd. This position gave me the opportunity to explore my two passions—English and medicine—by developing my editorial skills in the medical writing field. I am heavily involved in the orientation and training of new employees as well, which allows me to continue to use my educational skills."

High School

If you are contemplating a career as a writer or editor, you should take English, journalism, and communications courses in high school. Computer classes are also helpful. If you know in high school that you want to do medical or scientific writing or editing, it is to your advantage to take biology, physiology, chemistry, physics, math, health, and other science-related courses.

To get some hands-on experience, you should strongly consider working on your school newspaper or yearbook. You might want to volunteer to write a science column for your school paper, reporting on what you're learning in science class. If you can find no opportunities for medical or science writing, then writing of any kind will be beneficial.

Part-time employment at health care facilities, newspapers, publishing companies, or scientific research facilities can also provide training, background information, and insight that can be beneficial in this career. Volunteer opportunities are usually available in hospitals and nursing homes as well.

Postsecondary Training

Although not all writers and editors are college-educated, today's jobs almost always require a bachelor's degree. Many writers and editors earn an undergraduate degree in English, journalism, or liberal arts and then obtain a master's degree in a communications field such as science, medical writing, or medical editing. A good liberal arts education is important since you are often required to have expertise in many subject areas.

Writers and editors with an undergraduate degree may choose to get a graduate degree in medical or science writing, medical or science editing, corporate communications, document

The Benefits of Association Membership

Professional associations provide key support and assistance to professionals as they advance in their careers. The American Medical Writers Association (AMWA) is one of the premier professional organizations for medical writers, editors, and other professionals in the field of biomedical communication. The editors of *What Can I Do Now?: Health Care* asked James Cozzarin, president-elect of AMWA, to tell us about his association and the benefits of membership:

"The American Medical Writers Association comprises more than 5,200 biomedical communicators, including writers, editors, freelancers, educators, and professionals involved in public relations, advertising, and marketing. As such, we benefit from the insights and experiences of such a diverse membership in our collaborative and collegial interactions, in our educational programming, in our national and local conferences, and through our various member communications programs, including our Web site (http://www.amwa.org), our online listservs and bulletin boards, and our quarterly publication, the AMWA Journal. I am quite proud of our educational program, which offers both core and advanced curriculum certificates indicative of professional development. Curriculum workshops are routinely offered at the various local/regional conferences across the United States and Canada, and we host a national conference annually, at which more than 100 workshops and other educational opportunities are offered to attendees from across North America and around the world. We regularly host more than 850 attendees from as many as 15 countries, many of whom attend year after year. What brings them? The opportunity to learn more about their craft, the opportunity to network with colleagues from around the globe, the opportunity to work together to improve personally and professionally and to advance the interests of the profession. AMWA has taught me a great deal over the years. I am proud to be a member, to hold both core and advanced curriculum certificates, to be a workshop leader, and to be an officer of the association. Through active participation in AMWA and in other organizations—such as the Board of Editors in the Life Sciences and the Council of Science Editors—I hope to give a little something back to the profession that I find so rewarding."

design, or a related program. Many medical writers have also earned their Ph.D. and/or M.D. degrees. An advanced degree may open doors to a prestigious career.

In addition to your classroom studies, you should write or edit whenever you can and keep copies of anything you're proud of, particularly if it has to do with medicine or science. These clips, whether published or not and whether on paper, in electronic format, or both, should be added to your portfolio to serve as samples of the kind of work you can do. They should demonstrate your skills and style as well as how you deal with difficult issues.

Certification or Licensing

Certification is not mandatory; however, certification programs are available from various organizations and institutions. The American Medical Writers Association offers educational workshops leading to core or advanced curriculum certificates; and the Board of Editors in the Life Sciences offers a certification program. Many employers look for one or the other of these as evidence of a commitment to ongoing professional development and mastery in the field.

Internships and Volunteerships

Internships afford an invaluable opportunity to make contacts in the field and are excellent ways to build your portfolio. You should investigate internship programs that give you experience in the communications department of a corporation, medical institution, or research facility. Some newspapers, magazines, and public relations firms also have internships that give you the opportunity to write or edit.

Employers in the communications field are usually interested in seeing samples of your published work assembled in an organized portfolio or scrapbook. Working on your college's magazine or newspaper staff can help you build a portfolio. Sometimes small, regional magazines also buy articles or assign short pieces to writers and editors.

WHO WILL HIRE ME?

A fair amount of experience is required to gain a high-level position in this field.

Most writers and editors start out in entry-level positions. These jobs may be listed with college career services offices, or you may apply directly to the employment departments of corporations, institutions, universities, research facilities, nonprofit organizations, and government facilities that hire medical and science writers and editors. Many firms now hire entry-level writers and editors directly upon application or recommendation of college professors and career services offices. Job ads in newspapers and trade journals are another source for jobs. Serving an internship in college can give you the advantage of knowing people who can give you personal recommendations.

You may need to begin your career as a junior writer or editor and work your way up. This usually involves library research, preparation of rough drafts for part or all of a report, cataloging, and other related tasks. These are generally carried on under the supervision of a senior writer or editor.

Many medical and science writers and editors enter the field after working in public relations departments, the medical profession, or science-related industries. They may use their skills to transfer to specialized writing or editing positions or they may take additional courses or graduate work that focuses on writing, editing, or documentation skills.

Pharmaceutical and drug companies, medical research institutions, government organizations, insurance companies, health care facilities, nonprofit organizations, manufacturers, chemical companies, medical publishers, medical associations, and other medical-related companies employ medical writers and editors.

Many medical and science writers and editors are employed, often on a freelance basis, by newspapers, magazines, and the broadcast industries as well. Internet publishing is a growing field that hires these professionals. Corporations that deal with the medical or science industries also hire specialty writers and editors as their public information officers or to head up communications departments within their facilities.

WHERE CAN I GO FROM HERE?

Some writers enjoy writing so much that they simply continue to write and become recognized experts in their field. Their writings may come to be in demand by trade journals, newspapers, magazines, and the broadcast industry. Many experienced medical and science writers are promoted to head writing, documentation, or public relations departments within corporations or institutions. Others may move into managerial positions, perhaps becoming managing editor of a trade journal or magazine or director of publications at a university.

In book publishing houses, employees who start as editorial assistants or proofreaders and show promise generally become copy editors. After gaining skill in that position, they may be given a wider range of duties while retaining the same title. The next step may be a position as a *senior copy editor*, which involves over-seeing the work of junior copy editors, or as a *project editor*. The project editor performs a wide variety of tasks, including copyediting, coordinating the work of in-house and freelance copy editors, and managing the schedule of a particular project. From this position, an editor may move up to become *first assistant editor*, then *managing editor*, then *editor-in-chief*. These positions involve more management and decision making than is usually found in the positions described previously. The editor-in-chief works with the publisher to ensure that a suitable editorial policy is being followed, while the managing editor is responsible for all aspects of the editorial department. The assistant editor provides support to the managing editor.

Newspaper editors generally begin working on the copy desk, where they progress from less significant stories and projects to major news and feature stories. A common route to advancement is for copy editors to be promoted to a particular department, where they may move up the ranks to management positions. An editor who has achieved success in a department may become a *city editor*, who is responsible for news, or a managing editor, who runs the entire editorial operation of a newspaper.

The advancement path for magazine editors is similar to that of book editors. After they become copy editors, they work their way up to become senior editors, managing editors, and editors-in-chief. In many cases, magazine editors advance by moving from a position on one magazine to the same position with a larger or more prestigious magazine. Such moves often bring significant increases in both pay and status.

Freelance writers and editors who prove themselves and work successfully with clients may be able to demand increased contract fees or higher hourly rates.

James plans to continue advancing in his career at ProEd over the next decade. "ProEd is on the cutting edge of medical marketing," he says, "with robust and developing programs in continuing professional education, regulatory submission documentation support, and U.S. Food and Drug Administration advisory committee presentation support. As such, we are growing and expanding our staff. I see our editorial services team growing as well, and I plan to stay right here in the thick of things. Where do I see myself in the next 5 to 10 years? I hope to become director of the team, establishing myself in the position where I can best help to grow and shape the team and company to meet the new challenges that lay before us."

WHAT ARE THE SALARY RANGES?

Average salaries for writers/editors in medical communications ranged from $57,800 to $87,400 in 2004, depending on their employer and job duties, according to the American Medical Writers Association. The U.S. Department of Labor reports that writers and authors employed in all fields earned salaries that ranged from less than $23,700 to $87,660 or more in 2004. Editors earned salaries that

Related Jobs

- columnists
- foreign correspondents
- lexicographers
- newswriters
- public relations specialists
- reporters
- research assistants
- screenwriters
- technical writers and editors

ranged from less than $26,490 to $82,070 or more. Those employed in newspaper, book, and directory publishing had mean annual earnings of $50,210.

Earnings for freelance writers and editors vary depending on their expertise, reputation, and the kinds of articles they are contracted to write or edit. Rates may be paid by the piece, hourly, or per word.

Most full-time positions offer benefits such as insurance, sick leave, and paid vacation. Some jobs also provide tuition reimbursement and retirement benefits. Freelance writers and editors must pay for their own insurance; however, certain professional associations offer group insurance rates for members.

WHAT IS THE JOB OUTLOOK?

According to the U.S. Department of Labor, strong competition exists for writing and editing jobs. Continuing advances in medicine and science will create a demand for skilled writers and editors to interpret and relay that information to the public and other professionals. The daily developments in biotechnology, for example, such as tissue engineering, stem cell research, genetic therapies, and cancer vaccines, suggest that there will be plenty of topics to write about in future.

"In a domestic and global economy where jobs are increasingly scarce, you would be fortunate indeed to align yourself with a growth industry," says James. "I have been so fortunate, as the medical communications field appears to be doing well. As a medical editor, I will have work as long as medical writers continue to write. Medical writers will continue to write as long as science continues to develop new treatments for patients. It is the medical writer who works in concert with the clinician or investigator who has run a clinical trial to put the results of that research onto paper. It is the medical editor who helps the writer craft that information into a clear and concise message easily understood by the target audience. Together, we help put the latest information before the public eye, so that more informed choices can be made by physicians in the way they treat their patients, and so that sick people can get better, quicker. With this as the goal of the industry, the future employment outlook seems bright indeed."

Nurse Assistants

SUMMARY

Definition
Nurse assistants care for patients in hospitals, nursing homes, and other settings under the supervision of nurses.

Alternative Job Titles
Career nurse (or nursing) assistants (or aides)
Hospital attendants
Nurse or nursing aides
Nursing assistants
Orderlies

Salary Range
$15,400 to $21,220 to $29,520+

Educational Requirements
High school diploma; completion of training program in either a community college or vocational school

Certification or Licensing
Voluntary for hospitals
Required for nursing homes

Employment Outlook
Much faster than the average

High School Subjects
Anatomy and physiology
Biology
English (writing/literature)
Health
Sociology

Personal Interests
Helping people: emotionally
Helping people: physical health/medicine

Helping nursing home residents get showered, dressed, and off to breakfast, then taking residents to the bathroom—it had been a hectic morning and now Pam Owens must make a bed. It may not seem like a large task, but the resident is bedridden and fragile and can't be moved about much. Pam will leave the resident in the bed while making it; she'll work slowly and carefully, a contrast from the fast action that's been required of her all morning.

First, Pam draws the curtain to protect the resident's privacy. "Are you comfortable, Mrs. Smith?" she asks, adjusting the pillow and raising the bed. When she's certain that the resident is at ease and unexposed, she lowers the side rail and begins to make up half the bed. She then raises the side rail again and helps the resident to the other side of the bed to finish. Before leaving, she checks again with Mrs. Smith to make certain she's comfortable and has everything she needs. Mrs. Smith responds with a smile and she squeezes Pam's hand. Pam leaves the room with the certainty that her tasks are important to the residents and the facility.

WHAT DOES A NURSE ASSISTANT DO?

Though the job title suggests someone who assists nurses, *nurse assistants* actually perform many duties independently; in some cases, they become more closely involved with patients or nursing home residents than do registered nurses or licensed practical nurses. Nurse assistants work under the supervision of nurses and perform tasks that allow the nursing staff to perform their primary duties effectively and efficiently.

Nurse assistants perform basic nursing care in hospitals and nursing homes. Male nurse assistants are perhaps better known as *orderlies.* Working independently and alongside nurses and doctors, nurse assistants help move patients, assist in patients' exercise and nutrition, and see to the patients' personal hygiene. They bring the patients their meal trays and help them to eat. They push the patients on stretchers and in wheelchairs to operating and X-ray rooms. They also help to admit and discharge patients. Nurse assistants must keep charts of their work for review by nurses.

About 40 percent of the nurse assistants today work in nursing homes, tending to the daily care of elderly residents. They help residents with baths and showers, meals, and exercise. They help them in and out of their beds and to and from the bathroom. They also record the health of residents by taking body temperatures and checking blood pressures.

Because the residents are living within such close proximity to each other, and because they need help with personal hygiene and health care, a nurse assistant also takes care to protect the privacy of the resident. It is the responsibility of a nurse assistant to make the resident feel as comfortable as possible. Nurse assistants may also work with patients who are not fully functional, teaching them how to care for themselves, educating them in personal hygiene and health care.

The work can be strenuous, requiring the lifting and moving of patients. Nurse assistants must work with partners, or in groups, when performing the more strenuous tasks, so that neither the nurse assistant nor the resident is injured. Some requirements of the job can be as routine as changing sheets and helping a resident with phone calls, while other requirements can be as difficult and unattractive as assisting a resident with elimination and cleaning up a resident who has vomited.

Nurse assistants may be called upon by nurses and physicians to perform the more menial and unappealing tasks, but they also have the opportunity to develop meaningful relationships with residents. Nurse assistants work closely with residents, often gaining their trust and admiration. When residents are having personal problems, or problems with the staff, they may turn to the nurse assistant for help.

Nurse assistants generally work a 40-hour workweek, with some overtime. The hours and weekly schedule may be irregular, however, depending on the needs of the care institution. An assistant may have one day off in the middle of the week, followed by three days of work, then

Lingo to Learn

ambulatory care Serving patients who are able to walk.

acute care Providing emergency services and general medical and surgical treatment for acute disorders rather than long-term care.

asepsis Methods of sterilization to ensure the absence of germs.

gerontology A branch of medicine that deals with aging and the problems of the aged.

neonatal Pertaining to newborn children.

pediatrics A branch of medicine concerned with the development, care, and diseases of babies and children.

another day off. Nurse assistants are needed around the clock, so beginning assistants may be required to work late at night or very early in the morning.

WHAT IS IT LIKE TO BE A NURSE ASSISTANT?

Pam Owens works in a 120-bed long-term care facility in Winterhaven, Florida. She cares for patients with cancer, Alzheimer's, dementia, and other illnesses and diseases; patients who are recuperating from fractured hips, knee replacements, and car accidents; hospice patients; and those who may simply have no other place to go. She works under the supervision of registered nurses and licensed practical nurses. She also works with occupational therapists, physical therapists, and dietitians. But mostly she performs her own set of daily responsibilities.

"I start at 7:00 A.M.," Pam says, "and check all my patients, make sure they are all OK, make sure they all have a washcloth and towel, and take them to the washroom if they need to go. After that, I serve them breakfast, help them get dressed, and take them to therapy."

In addition to caring for patients during the day, Pam must attend to call lights; call lights are the way residents signal the nurse assistants for help. "We are supposed to respond to call lights in a reasonable amount of time—in our facility this is within one to three minutes," she explains. "These go off all day and all night."

At the end of her workday, Pam fills out daily activity sheets for each patient that she cared for. The activity sheets are part of a patient's chart, and doctors and nurses review them to learn more about the status of a patient. "I record," explains Pam, "whether I gave patients a bath or shower, how much I had to help them get dressed, their bowel movements, the percentage of food they ate (the dietitian uses this information to monitor and develop nutritional treatment plans), their vital signs, whether they were continent or incontinent, and other information. I am the eyes and ears for my nurse, and I report anything that I see that is not status quo with the patient." The daily activity sheets are considered legal documents and may be reviewed by state inspectors if any legal questions arise as to the care of a patient. Pam spends about 30 minutes preparing the day's activity sheets.

To Be a Successful Nurse Assistant, You Should . . .

- be a compassionate person
- be in good health
- be able to perform some heavy lifting
- have a great deal of patience
- take orders well
- be a good team player
- be emotionally stable

Pam's day is usually complete at 3:00 P.M., though she occasionally works overtime. "Every now and then, a person might call in sick, and I might stay till 5:00, but that doesn't happen too often."

DO I HAVE WHAT IT TAKES TO BE A NURSE ASSISTANT?

A nurse assistant must care about the work and the patients and must show a general understanding and compassion for the ill, disabled, and the elderly. "You need to have compassion and a love of your job," Pam Owens says. "Otherwise, there is no sense in being a nurse assistant."

Renee Hollowell, a nurse assistant in hospice care, says that the loss of independence and privacy is the most devastating part of being ill. "Helping with meals or laundry is a given in this profession, but to assist with personal care, you have to have a great respect for patients in order to provide appropriate and sensitive care."

Because of the rigorous physical demands placed on a nurse assistant, you should be in good health. Also, the hours and responsibilities of the job won't allow you to take many sick days. Along with this good physical health, you should have good mental health, as well. The job can be emotionally demanding, requiring your patience and stability. You should also be able to take orders and to work as part of a team.

Though the work can often be rewarding, a nurse assistant must also be prepared for the worst. "Dealing with difficult persons, for example, an Alzheimer's or dementia patient, can be very challenging," Pam says. "They may not want to get dressed or eat. They may be verbally abusive, and some of them like to hit. You just have to love them. If you don't love them, you're not going to be able to follow through with your care and get them to do what you want them to do."

Nurse assistants also need to have pride in their work. "You have to be able to look at yourself," explains Pam, "and say 'this is a job that I love to do, and this is my career and I'm proud of it.'"

HOW DO I BECOME A NURSE ASSISTANT?
Education
High School

Communication skills are valuable for a nurse assistant, so take English, speech, and writing courses. Science courses, such as biology and anatomy, will also prepare you for future training. Renee Hollowell encourages students to take courses in health, but also those that help them learn about death and dying since nurse assistants—especially those working in hospice care—care for patients who are gravely ill or dying.

Postsecondary Training

Nurse assistants are not required to have a college degree but may have to complete a short training course at a community college or vocational school. These training courses, usually instructed by a registered nurse, teach basic nursing skills and prepare students for the state certification exam. Nurse assistants typically begin the training courses after getting their first job as an assistant, and the course work is incorporated into their on-the-job training.

Many people work as nurse assistants as they pursue other medical professions; someone interested in becoming a nurse or a paramedic may work as an assistant while taking courses. A high school student or a student in a premedical program may work as a nurse assistant part-time before going on to medical school.

Certification or Licensing

Nurse assistants in hospitals are not required to be certified, but those working in nursing homes must pass a state exam. The Omnibus Budget Reconciliation Act (OBRA), passed by Congress in 1987, requires nursing homes to hire only certified nurse assistants.

OBRA also requires continuing education for nurse assistants, and periodic evaluations.

Pam Owens became a certified nursing assistant by taking and passing a written test. Today, nurse assistants must take a hands-on test to become certified. "They must demonstrate skills," Pam says, "such as how to give a bath, dress or undress a patient, take blood pressure, transfer people in and out of beds, and other tasks that nurse assistants are expected to perform." Pam feels that certification is a good thing because many aspiring nurse assistants have never been caregivers or taken care of patients and need to learn appropriate skills before they are trusted with the care of a patient. To maintain her certification in Florida, Pam must complete 18 hours of continuing education annually.

Internships and Volunteerships

Because a high school diploma is not required of nurse assistants, many high school students are hired by nursing homes and hospitals for part-time work. Job opportunities may also exist in a hospital or nursing home kitchen, introducing you to diet and nutrition, as well as in nursing home activity departments. Also, volunteer work can familiarize you with the work nurses and nurse assistants perform, as well as introduce you to some medical terminology.

WHO WILL HIRE ME

Approximately 42 percent of all nurse assistants work in nursing care facilities.

Other places where they are employed include hospitals, halfway houses, retirement centers, and private homes.

Because of the high demand for nurse assistants, you can apply directly to the health care facilities in your area. Most will probably have a human resources department that advertises positions in the newspaper and interviews applicants.

WHERE CAN I GO FROM HERE?

For the most part, there is not much opportunity for advancement within the job of nurse assistant. To move up in a health care facility requires additional training. Some nurse assistants, after gaining experience and learning medical technology, enroll in nursing programs, or may even decide to pursue medical degrees or opportunities in health care management. Lori Porter worked as a certified nursing assistant for seven years before becoming a nursing home administrator. She also co-founded the National Association of Geriatric Nursing Assistants (NAGNA), the first and only national professional association for nursing assistants in the United States. "I am responsible for the oversight of the association as a whole, membership, operations, education, public policy agenda, and a variety of other tasks," she explains. "I represent the association on a national front through public speaking and negotiating with long-term-care health provider's to partner with NAGNA to serve the needs of their CNAs [certified nurse assistants]."

A nursing home requires a lot of hard work and dedication so nurse assistants frequently burn out or quit before completing their training. Others may choose another aspect of the job, such as working as a home health aide. Helping patients in their homes, these aides see to the client's personal health, hygiene, and home care.

WHAT ARE THE SALARY RANGES?

Although the salaries for most health care professionals vary by region and population, the average hourly wage of nurse assistants is about the same across the country. Midwestern states and less populated areas, where a large staff of nurse assistants may be needed to make up for a smaller staff of nurses and therapists, may pay a little more per hour.

According to the U.S. Department of Labor, nurse assistants earned median hourly wages of $10.20 in 2004. For full-time work at 40 hours per week, this hourly wage translates into a yearly income of approximately $21,220. The lowest paid 10 percent earned less than $7.40 per hour (approximately $15,400 per year), and the highest paid 10 percent earned more than $14.19 per hour (approximately $29,520 annually).

Benefits are usually based on the hours worked, length of employment, and the policies of the facility. Some offer paid vacation and holidays, medical or hospital insurance, and retirement plans. Some also provide free meals to their workers.

Related Jobs

- ambulance attendants
- child care attendants
- emergency medical technicians
- home health aides
- morgue attendants
- occupational therapy aides
- optometric assistants
- perfusionists
- physical therapy aides
- psychiatric aides
- surgical technicians

WHAT IS THE JOB OUTLOOK?

Lori Porter sees a very bright employment future for nursing assistants. "Nurse assisting offers a career freedom rarely found in America," she says. "Once certified, a nurse assistant can go anywhere in the United States and find a position in their chosen field within 24 hours. This level of freedom is priceless. The largest growing demographic is geriatrics and, therefore, long-term care offers unlimited opportunities in health care professional growth. Hospital acute care is often depicted as more exciting or prestigious, but those working in long-term care often find their work more challenging and rewarding. I highly recommend the profession in general, but certainly recommend long-term care specifically."

There will continue to be many job opportunities for nurse assistants. Because of the physical and emotional demands of the job, and because of the lack of advancement opportunities, there is a high turnover rate of employees. Also, health care is constantly changing; more opportunities open for nurse assistants as different kinds of health care facilities are developed. Business-based health organizations are limiting the services of health care professionals and looking for cheaper ways to provide care. This may provide opportunities for those looking for work as nurse assistants.

Government and private agencies are also developing more programs to assist dependent people. And as the number of people 65-years-of-age and older continues to rise, new and larger nursing care facilities will be needed.

Nurses

SUMMARY

Definition
Nurses administer medical care to sick or injured individuals and help people achieve health and prevent disease.

Alternative Job Title
Staff nurses

Salary Range
$24,910 to $53,640 to $77,170+

Educational Requirements
Varies by position

Certification or Licensing
Required for certain specialties (certification)
Required (licensing)

Employment Outlook
About as fast as the average (licensed practical nurses)
Much faster than the average (registered nurses)

High School Subjects
Anatomy and physiology
Biology
Chemistry
Health
Mathematics

Personal Interests
Helping people: emotionally
Helping people: physical health/medicine
Science

It's three in the morning in the intensive care unit. Nurses on the night shift are making their rounds, listening to the instruments that monitor their patients, changing IV bags, or giving medicine. In the emergency room several cases come in all at once; even though they are seven hours into their shift, the trauma nurses immediately snap to in a flurry of activity. Their ability to react quickly and make decisions under pressure can make the difference between life and death.

Meanwhile, at a retirement community not far away, a live-in nurse assists her client to the bathroom, walking slowly to help her navigate the long hallway from her bedroom safely. Although it is 11:00 o'clock at night, the nurse shows no hint of irritation or fatigue. It is her job to help her patient in any way she can.

WHAT DO NURSES DO?

Just as the title "doctor" encompasses numerous specialties and branches of study, the title *nurse* is an umbrella term, covering many different aspects of nursing. Although nurses work in various health care facilities, they have three basic goals: to assist the ill, disabled, or elderly in the recovery or maintenance of life functions; to prevent illness and relapse of illness; and to promote health in the community. Most nurses come into contact with patients more frequently than other members of the health care community. Doctors are busy with diagnosis and the creation of treatment plans, and often do not have time to carry out the plans themselves. Because of this, nurses often provide the human element in a patient's treatment. They observe a patient's symptoms and evaluate progress or lack of progress. Nurses are also responsible for educating their patients and families on how to cope with a long-term illness or disability.

The field of nursing is broken down by the setting in which a nurse works. A *registered nurse* typically works under the guidance of a physician, who will develop a care plan for a patient that the nurse helps to administer. But the specific work of each nurse can take many forms. *General duty nurses* offer bedside nursing care and observe the progress of the patients. They may also supervise *licensed practical nurses* (who perform many of the general duties of nursing and may be responsible for some clerical duties) and aides. *Surgical nurses* are part of a logistical team in the operating room that supports the surgeon. They sterilize instruments, prepare patients for surgery, and coordinate the transfer of patients to and from the operating room. A *maternity nurse,* or *neonatal nurse,* looks after newborn infants, assists in the delivery room, and educates new mothers and fathers on basic childcare. A *head nurse* directs and coordinates the activities of the nursing staff. Other hospital staff

nurses are trained to work in intensive care units, the emergency room, and in the pediatric ward.

Heading up the entire nursing program in the hospital is the *nursing service director,* who administers the nursing program to maintain standards of patient care. The nursing service director advises the medical staff, department heads, and the hospital administrator in matters relating to nursing services and helps prepare the department budget.

Nurses work in varied settings. *Home health nurses* provide nursing care, prescribed by a physician, to patients at home. They assist a wide range of patients, such as those recovering from illnesses and accidents, and must be able to work independently. *Private duty nurses* may work in hospitals or in a patient's home. They are employed by the patient they are caring for or by the patient's family. Their duties are carried out in cooperation with the patient's physician.

Office nurses work in clinics or at the private practice of a physician. Their duties may combine nursing skills—taking blood pressure, assisting with outpatient procedures, patient education—with administrative or office duties such as scheduling appointments, keeping files, and answering phones. Nurses in this field may work for a health maintenance organization (HMO) or an insurance company.

Nursing home nurses direct the care of residents in long-term care facilities. The work is similar to that done in hospitals; however, a nursing home nurse cares for patients with conditions ranging from a hip fracture to Parkinson's disease. *Public health nurses,* or *community health nurses,* work with government and private agencies to educate the public about health care issues. Their work might include creating a community blood pressure testing site, speaking about nutrition and disease, and providing immunizations and disease screenings for members of their community. Many school children are screened by *public health nurses,* or *school nurses,* for such conditions as poor vision and scoliosis.

Occupational health nurses, or *industrial nurses,* provide nursing care in a clinic at a work site. They provide emergency care, work on accident prevention programs, and offer health counseling.

Administrators in the community health field include nursing directors, educational directors, and nursing supervisors. Some nurses go into nursing education and work with nursing students to instruct them on theories and skills they will need to enter the profession. *Nursing instructors* may give classroom instruction and demonstrations or supervise nursing students on hospital units. Some instructors eventually become nursing school directors, university faculty, or deans of a university degree program. Nurses also have the opportunity to direct staff development and continuing education programs for nursing personnel in hospitals.

Advanced practice nurses are nurses with training beyond the requirements for the RN designation. There are four primary categories of nurses included in this category: *nurse-midwives, clinical nurse specialists, nurse anesthetists,* and *nurse practitioners.*

Nurse-midwives are registered nurses with advanced training who assist in family planning, pregnancy, and childbirth. They also provide routine health care for women. Clinical nurse specialists (CNSs) have completed advanced clinical nurses' educational practice requirements. Qualified to handle a wide variety of physical and mental health problems, CNSs are primarily involved in providing primary health care and psychotherapy.

Nurse anesthetists, also known as *certified registered nurse anesthetists,* have advanced training in anesthesiology. They are responsible for administering, supervising, and monitoring anesthesia-related care for patients undergoing surgical procedures. General anesthesia is not necessary for all surgical procedures; therefore, nurse anesthetists also work on cases in which they provide various types of local anesthesia—topical, infiltration, nerve block, spinal, and epidural or caudal.

Nurse practitioners have advanced training and education that enables them to carry out many of the responsibilities traditionally handled by physicians. Some nurse practitioners specialize in a certain field, such as pediatrics, oncology, critical care, or primary care. The most common specialty is a *family nurse practitioner,* who usually serves community-based health clinics.

Some nurses are consultants to hospitals, nursing schools, industrial organizations, and public health agencies. They advise clients on such administrative matters as staff organization, nursing techniques, curricula, and education programs. Other administrative specialists include educational directors for the state board of nursing, who are concerned with maintaining well-defined educational standards, and executive directors of professional nurses' associations, who administer programs developed by the board of directors and the members of the association.

Some nurses choose to enter the armed forces. All types of nurses, except private duty nurses, are represented in the military services. They provide skilled nursing care to active-duty and retired members of the armed forces and their families. In addition to basic nursing skills, military nurses are trained to provide care in various environments, including field hospitals, on-air evacuation flights, and onboard ships. Military nurses actively influence the development of health care through nursing research. Advances influenced by military nurses include the development of the artificial kidney (dialysis unit) and the concept of the intensive care unit.

WHAT IS IT LIKE TO BE A NURSE?

Jim Raper has been an administrative director and a nurse practitioner in the University of Alabama-Birmingham (UAB) Outpatient HIV/AIDS Clinic for the past 11 years. He is also a research assistant professor of medicine and clinical assistant professor of nursing at UAB. In addition to these positions, Jim has worked as director of emergency and ambulatory services at Butterworth Hos-

---

Lingo to Learn

case manager A nurse or administrator who coordinates the medical care of a patient.

crash cart The cart that carries medicines, equipment, and machines that may be needed in an emergency situation in an intensive care unit or emergency room.

extubate To remove a breathing tube from a patient

intubate To insert breathing apparatus into the throat of a patient who is unable to breathe satisfactorily.

nursing home A long-term care facility that provides the elderly and chronically ill with health care and assistance with daily activities, such as bathing, eating, and dressing.

skilled nursing facility A facility that provides round-the-clock medical care by registered nurses and other licensed health care professionals.

vital signs The temperature, pulse rate, breathing rate, blood pressure, and level of pain of a patient.

---

pital in Grand Rapids, Michigan, and held a number of other positions at UAB including hospital night administrator, emergency department nurse manager, and cardiovascular operating room charge nurse. "I became a nurse on the advice of a female nurse who was one of my high school teachers," he says. "She knew I was one of six children from a home of very modest means. She knew of my interest in health care and encouraged me to pursue nursing as an 'introduction' into the health sciences. Once I started my career in nursing I just kept pushing forward. Nursing has afforded me with a great profession. I work with some of the best and brightest people in the world. I'm always challenged to push myself, to expand my abilities, to maximize my potential. I serve people in need while I gain personal and professional fulfillment. I laugh and cry as I experience the lives of the patients to whom I provide care."

Jim begins his day around 6:30 A.M. He typically works 12 hours a day, five days a week. "That's my choice," he says. "I find great personal and professional fulfillment in what I am accomplishing." Jim says that he wears many hats throughout the course of his workday. "The variety of work is one of the things I find so exciting about what I do," he says. "When I get to work I put on my administration hat. I begin by physically checking out the clinic to be sure everything is ready for the activities of the day. I review the billing statements from the activities of the previous day, review my patients' laboratory and other test results, and check voice messages and e-mails for matters of importance before patients start arriving at 8:00 A.M."

At this time, Jim says he begins his nurse practitioner duties, meeting with patients as they begin to arrive. "I'm responsible for performing clinical (diagnostic/therapeutic) functions and procedures," he says, "as appropriate to my scope of preparation as a mid-level medical provider and specialty certification. I take care of patients along a very broad

continuum of health. Some are just coming for routine examinations and others are gravely ill, near death, with many complex problems. I am able to help heal many of my patients. But, some are too sick to get well. Eventually they die. I always try to be there for them. I play a very active role in helping my patients live the best possible lives and not suffer when it is time to die."

In addition to the aforementioned responsibilities, Jim also works with students of all varieties (e.g., medical, nursing, pharmacy, interns, residents, and fellows). "This is when I put on my educator hat," he says. "I almost always serve as a preceptor to graduate students in the various nurse practitioner programs at UAB. Wearing my researcher hat is also very rewarding. Mostly I'm involved with clinical trails and outcomes research in the field of HIV/AIDS."

Kevin Daugherty Hook has worked as a registered nurse for seven years. When he first began working in the field, he worked the evening shift at Mt. Sinai Hospital in New York City, on the telemetry unit. He then moved to Indianapolis, Indiana, and worked for Clarian Health Partners, Methodist Hospital, in the Cardiac Comprehensive Critical Care Unit for six years. "I was always interested in medicine and/or nursing, even when I was in high school," he says. "I had so many interests that the thought of going through the rigors of medical school to the exclusion of all my other interests didn't sound interesting. Although I considered nursing school the first time I went to college, the year was 1974 and I didn't know any male nurses at the time. I think the stigma attached to men in nursing kept me away for a very long time."

Kevin begins his workday by getting reports on his patients from the nurse on the previous shift. "While the nurse is describing the patients," he says, "I formulate a plan in my head about the priorities for each patient, and, in fact, which patient may be a priority. While all my patients deserve my best, the reality is some are sicker than others and need a lot more nursing care. Kevin's main responsibilities for each patient are to perform physical assessments, administer medications, and provide ongoing monitoring throughout the day. "I need to know when to get a physician involved in some problem and when the problem is pretty much a nursing problem and take care of it myself."

Secondary issues that Kevin must address during the day include dealing with family stress, educating patients, keeping the medical team informed about significant changes in the patient's status, and arranging for transportation when patients are leaving the unit for tests such as CT scans and MRIs.

DO I HAVE WHAT IT TAKES TO BE A REGISTERED NURSE?

You should enjoy working with people, especially those who may experience fear or anger because of an illness. Patience, compassion, and calmness are qualities needed by anyone working in this career. In addition, you must be able to give directions as well as follow instructions and work as part of a health care team. Anyone interested in becoming a registered nurse should also have a strong desire to continue learning because new tests, procedures, and technologies are constantly being developed for the medical world.

Nurses must also be able to manage patient information and be able to convey it effectively to other nurses, physicians, and other health care professionals. "Nurses are really the information managers about patients to all the other members of the team, as well as to the family of the patient," says Kevin Daugherty Hook. "All information about patients, from their physical and emotional status, to pertinent labs that need to be responded to, flows through the nurse. If you want to know about a patient, ask the nurse."

More than anything else, nurses must be genuinely concerned for their patients. They must be advocate for their patients and ensure that they are receiving the best possible care.

To Be a Successful Nurse, You Should . . .

- have keen observational skills
- be able to work under pressure
- follow orders precisely
- be well organized
- be caring and sympathetic
- handle emergencies calmly

HOW DO I BECOME A REGISTERED NURSE?

Education

Jim Raper earned a bachelor of science in nursing from Kent State University, and then served three years in the U.S. Army Nurse Corps (ANC). While an officer in the ANC, and stationed at Redstone Arsenal in Alabama, Jim enrolled in graduate school at the University of Alabama-Huntsville, where he received a master of science in nursing. He then worked for five years before beginning the next phase of his education—eventually earning a doctor of science in nursing, a post-masters family nurse practitioner certificate, and a juris doctorate. "Obviously, I like school," Jim says.

Kevin Daugherty Hook came to nursing as a second career. "Before becoming a nurse," he says, "I taught high school English for two years and completed a master's degree at Indiana University in religious studies and ethics. Columbia University in New York, as well as the University of Pennsylvania and many other universities, have a fast-track bachelor's degree in nursing designed for men and women who already have degrees in other areas. So I completed the accelerated BSN program at Columbia University, worked for several years, and am now a student in the graduate program at the University of Pennsylvania to become an adult and gerontological nurse practitioner."

High School

If you are interested in becoming a nurse, you should take high school mathematics and science courses, including biology, chemistry, and physics. Health courses will also be helpful. English and speech courses should not be neglected because you must be able to communicate well with patients.

Postsecondary Training

Those interested in a career as a licensed practical nurse usually enroll in a practical nursing program after graduating from high school. There are about 1,100 state-approved programs in the United States that provide practical nursing training. Most programs last 12 months, with time spent for both classroom study and supervised clinical care. Courses include basic nursing concepts, anatomy, physiology, medical-surgical nursing, pediatrics, obstetrics, nutrition, and first aid. Clinical practice is most often in a hospital setting.

There are three training programs for registered nurses: associate's degree programs, diploma programs, and bachelor's degree programs. All three programs combine classroom education with actual nursing experience. Associate degrees in nursing usually involve a two-year program at a junior or community college that is affiliated with a hospital. Many associate's degree nurses seek further schooling in bachelor's programs after they have found employment in order to take advantage of tuition reimbursement programs.

The diploma program is conducted through independent nursing schools and teaching hospitals and usually lasts three years.

A bachelor's degree is recommended for nurses who must compete in an era of cutbacks and small staffs. Additionally, bachelor's degree programs are recommended for those who may want to go into administration or supervision. It is also required for jobs in public health agencies and for admission to graduate school.

Nurses who are interested in becoming advanced practice nurses, nurse managers, or nurse educators typically earn graduate degrees.

Certification or Licensing

The National Federation of Licensed Practical Nurses offers voluntary certifi-

Nursing Pros and Cons

Nursing, like any other profession, has its plusses and minuses. The editors of *What Can I Do Now?: Health Care* asked Kevin Daugherty Hook to tell us what he likes best and least about his career.

"The pros of nursing are that nursing calls on all skill sets: intellectual, emotional, organizational, and clinical. Nurses are always in demand; but now, more importantly, nursing provides an amazing array of career trajectories, from bedside, to teaching, to administration and/or research, and now, increasingly, advanced practice nursing such as nurse practitioners.

The cons are changing for the better, but hospitals still treat nurses as second-class citizens a lot of the time, and physicians don't always treat nurses as vital members of the team caring for the patient. I think a lot of this is generational and will pass away with time."

cation for LPNs who specialize in IV therapy or gerontology. Contact the federation for more information.

Certification for registered nurses is available to those who work in specific specialties, such as school nursing and nurse practitioners. Contact the professional association (see the "Look to the Pros" chapter) that represents nurses in the field in which you are interested for more information.

After graduating from an approved school of practical nursing, licensed practical nursing candidates will need to pass an examination to become licensed. All states and the District of Columbia require practical nurses to be licensed and to renew that license every two years. The state board of nursing issues the practical nursing license (or the vocational nursing license in California and Texas) once the National Council Licensure Examination for Practical Nurses, a written exam, is passed. Legal minimum requirements for the license are set by each state through its board of nursing, so these may vary from state to state. Licensed practical nurses in one state wishing to practice nursing in another state must apply to the board of nursing in that state. Although requirements vary slightly, it is generally not difficult to obtain another license and may not even require a written examination. Licensed practical nurses can identify themselves by putting the initials "LPN" or "LVN" (in Texas and California) after their names.

Licensing for registered nurses is required in all 50 states, and license renewal or continuing education credits are also required periodically. In some cases, licensing in one state will automatically grant licensing in reciprocal states. For further information, contact your state's nursing board. (See the National Council of State Boards of Nursing Web site at http://www.ncsbn.org for contact information.)

You will need additional training if you wish to advance into specialized practices, administration, and teaching. This may include further clinical training within the hospital in an area such as pediatrics or gerontology, or entering a master's degree program.

Internships and Volunteerships

Nursing students are required to complete several nursing internships, or clinical rotations, as part of their postsecondary training. Depending on your educational program, your school may offer these opportunities on site or have agreements with nearby hospitals and medical centers. Rotations focus on specific practice areas such as oncology, geriatrics, surgery, or pediatrics.

It is possible to volunteer in many of the places nurses work, in order to decide if nursing is the career you want. Hospitals will take on high school volunteers as candy stripers or assistants, delivering mail and flowers, visiting with patients, and doing routine office work. While volunteerships at this level are not really concerned with patient treatment, they enable the prospective nurse to understand the way the hospital works and who is responsible for what duty.

While volunteering, you may be given more opportunity as a technician or as an aide to contribute to patient care. In many cases, if hospitals know you are seriously considering a career in nursing, they will give you better opportunities for hands-on involvement and experiences. Hospitals have a vested interest in training people to be nurses, especially if it means they will be able to hire somebody who is already familiar with the workings of their administration and setup.

WHO WILL HIRE ME?

Approximately 726,000 licensed practical nurses and 2.4 million registered nurses are employed in the United States. The most obvious place to look for a nursing job is in a hospital. Nurses also are needed in retirement communities, in government facilities, in schools, and in private practices. In fact, nursing in hospitals is not expected to grow as fast as other aspects of nursing, due to rising costs and a general trend away from inpatient care. The reductions caused by fewer available hospital jobs will be taken up by increased opportunities in newer fields. Insurance companies now hire nurses to assist in case management and to ensure that insured patients are getting the correct kind of care from their health care providers. One of the fastest-growing fields in nursing is home health care. Nurses who care for people on a part-time basis in their homes are in great demand for a variety of reasons. Technology has enabled many people to live free of health care institutions, but these people may still require assistance with some of their treatments.

Many surgical centers and emergency medical centers are taking the place of hospital emergency rooms. This will provide work for nurses who require a flexible schedule but who do not wish to work in a hospital. The number of older people with functional disabilities is growing, and jobs will be available in long-term care facilities for specialized conditions such as Alzheimer's disease.

Nurses should look in local newspapers and on the Internet for positions, in addition to contacting preferred employers to ask what they may have available. Many professional nursing associations offer job listings at their Web sites or in their professional journals and newsletters. Knowing where you would like to work, achieving educational credits in that field, and making sure those in charge of hiring know you are available are the key steps to finding a desirable nursing position.

WHERE CAN I GO FROM HERE?

Experienced nurses can advance in many ways. Those who want challenges beyond direct patient care may become teachers or administrators. Others continue their education and become clinical nurse specialists, nurse practitioners, certified nurse-midwives, or nurse anesthetists. Master's degrees and doctorates are required for many of these positions.

Five years from now, Jim Raper plans to continue to work in his current positions. "I love what I do," he says. "It's the perfect job. In 10 years I'll be approaching 60, and it may be difficult to keep up my current pace of life. I might switch over to full-time teaching at that point."

"I can't imagine not working," says Kevin Daugherty Hook, "so I don't see myself retiring even when I turn 65. I'd like to work as nurse practitioner for several years and gradually move my career into a consulting role, both in ethics and in clinical care."

WHAT ARE THE SALARY RANGES?

According to the U.S. Department of Labor, LPNs earned an average of $34,650 annually in 2004. Ten percent earned less than $24,910, and 10 percent earned more than $47,440. Nursing homes tend to pay a little more than hospitals. The mean annual salary of licensed practical nurses working full-time in nursing homes, excluding shift differentials, was $36,870 in 2004.

According to the U.S. Department of Labor, registered nurses had median annual earnings of $53,640 in 2004. Salaries ranged from less than $38,050 to more than $77,170. Earnings of RNs vary according to employer. Registered nurses who worked for employment services

Related Jobs

- paramedics
- physician assistants
- physicians
- psychiatric aides
- transplant coordinators

earned mean annual salaries of $64,700; those who worked at hospitals earned $56,630, and RNs who worked at nursing and personal care facilities earned $50,490.

Most health care employers provide a good benefits plan for their workers, as well as flexible work schedules, childcare, and bonuses. Educational incentives take the form of in-house training and tuition reimbursement, which can enable nurses to increase their skills and potential for advancement at no or little cost to themselves.

WHAT IS THE JOB OUTLOOK?

According to the U.S. Department of Labor, employment of LPNs is expected to increase about as fast as the average for all occupations in response to the needs of a rapidly growing older population and to the cost constraints hospitals experience relative to providing long-term patient care. As in most other occupations, replacement needs will be the main source of job openings. Much better employment opportunities are expected for LPNs employed in non-hospital settings. LPNs employed in physicians' offices and in outpatient care centers will enjoy faster than average growth. Those employed in home health care services will enjoy much faster than average growth.

Employment for registered nurses is expected to grow much faster than average, according to the U.S. Department of Labor. As the cost for medical specialists skyrockets, more general health care practitioners will be in demand for the services that they can provide at less cost. Nurse practitioners, for example, can diagnose, treat, and manage uncomplicated health problems.

Technological advances in patient care and the health care needs of an aging population have created a demand for skilled nurses in many areas. Ambulatory, home health, and outpatient care are expected to provide the most employment opportunities, while the need for nurses in hospitals will grow less rapidly. Nurses will be in high demand in nursing homes and in facilities that care for critically and terminally ill patients.

There are also many part-time job openings for nurses who do not want a full-time position.

Staying aware of trends in health care will give prospective nurses a good idea of the job market for their skills. Trade journals, association membership materials, and health-care laws all discuss the course that health care is taking today, and are valuable sources of information for predicting where the future demand in nursing will be.

Physical Therapists

SUMMARY

Definition
Physical therapists help alleviate pain, prevent disability, and restore mobility and function in patients with injuries, diseases, or birth defects. They also help improve the physical conditions of healthy people.

Alternative Job Title
Physiotherapists

Salary Range
$25,000 to $61,560 to $150,000+

Educational Requirements
Master's degree

Certification or Licensing
Recommended (certification)
Required by all states (licensing)

Outlook
Much faster than the average

High School Subjects
Anatomy and physiology
Biology
Health
Physical education

Personal Interests
Exercise/personal fitness
Helping people: emotionally
Helping people: physical health/medicine

One of physical therapist Jenni Masterson's favorite memories occurred when she was a student on a rehab hospital rotation treating a woman who had sustained a stroke. The woman had recently purchased an RV with her husband in anticipation of her retirement, and lamented her inability to climb the stairs to the RV.

"At the time," Jenni recalls, "she was using a wheelchair to get around and had little use of her right arm and leg because of weakness."

One day, after Jenni had finished helping the women walk in the parallel bars, she told her they would be trying something new. "I wheeled her chair over to a series of four steps and told her we were going to try to go up them. My patient didn't say anything, but eyed them with a look of disdain. I told her that I thought she was ready, and I knew she could go up and down those stairs with my help. With my help, and after about 10 minutes, she had gone up and down the stairs."

"I helped her sit back in the chair, and she began to sob uncontrollably. When I asked her what was wrong, she replied that she was crying because she had been looking at those stairs for weeks and thinking that if only she could learn to go up and down them again that maybe she could learn to go up and down her RV stairs and travel with her husband in their retirement. She went on to explain that she had come to think that it would never happen, but now she knew that it could happen and that was as good as having her life back. She taught me in 15 minutes what being a therapist is truly about—restoring function to a patient to enable them to do the things that are most important to them in life."

WHAT DOES A PHYSICAL THERAPIST DO?

Many illnesses, injuries, birth defects, and other health conditions can have a drastic effect on a person's mobility and overall quality of life. *Physical therapists* (PTs) work with patients to help to relieve their pain and restore them to full function, if possible, or to help them adjust to life after disabling illnesses or injuries so that they can live independent lives. Physical therapists work as part of a team of health care professionals, which may include general practitioners, specialists, radiologists, occupational therapists, and social workers.

A physical therapist first consults a patient's medical history. The physical therapist may then speak with the patient's physician to discuss the patient's health and treatment options. The physical therapist also speaks to the patient to learn about the kind and amount of pain the patient feels. The therapist seeks to identify aspects of the patient's behavior, activity, and lifestyle that cause an onset of pain.

The next step is to conduct clinical tests to measure the patient's strength, range of motion, and ability to function. The physical therapist may observe the patient as he or she performs certain tasks, such as walking up and down stairs, walking on a treadmill, bending and stretching, and lifting objects. Once the patient's problems have been identified, the physical therapist will discuss them with the patient and with a team of health care professionals in order to set treatment goals and design a plan that will help the patient accomplish these goals.

Treatment is specifically designed according to the patient's needs and abilities. A physical therapist treating a patient who is paralyzed or otherwise immobilized may begin with passive exercises, such as stretching and manipulating joints and muscles. The therapist may use electrical stimulation, hot or cold compresses, or ultrasound in order to stimulate muscles and relieve pain. Traction and deep-tissue massages can also help relieve a patient's pain and restore function. As treatment progresses, the therapist may design a program of movements and exercises that help the patient regain strength and mobility.

For certain patients, such as a person who has suffered a stroke or lost a limb, a return to full function is not possible. Physical therapists work with such patients to help them adjust to their new conditions. They may help a patient adapt to wearing a prosthetic device, such as an artificial limb, or to using crutches or a wheelchair. Other patients must relearn certain activities, such as walking, dressing, and climbing in and out of bathtubs, in order to return to independent lives. Physical therapists work with cardiac patients to increase their endurance and minimize the risk of further heart problems. Burn patients require treatment that will reduce scarring and help them maintain flexibility.

Physical therapists also work with athletes and other people who seek to improve their physical conditions. A physical therapist may devise an exercise program designed to enhance a person's athletic performance. The therapist will observe the person's movements and suggest ways of improving posture and technique to achieve the person's goals. Other professionals besides physical therapists who do this type of work include athletic trainers, personal trainers, and physical instructors.

The American Physical Therapy Association recognizes seven specialty areas within physical therapy: cardiopulmonary, clinical electrophysiology, geriatrics, neurology, orthopedics, pediatrics, and sports physical therapy.

WHAT IS IT LIKE TO BE A PHYSICAL THERAPIST?

Jenni Masterson has been a physical therapist for five years and a certified athletic trainer for nine years. She works for Novacare Rehabilitation, a national company that provides outpatient physical, occupational, and speech therapy. "When I was in high school," she recalls, "I had an interest in science courses, especially anatomy and physiology. I knew I was interested in a health field, but did not settle on a specific discipline until after volunteering as a student athletic trainer at my high school and attending some physical therapy appointments with my father, who had rotator cuff tendonitis. After these experiences, it was clear to me that physical therapy was an exciting career opportunity where the practitioner was able to see the positive effect their treatments had on a

---

Lingo to Learn

modalities The various technical procedures used in physical therapy during treatment. They include the following:

cryotherapy The therapeutic use of cold.

diathermy The production of heat in parts of the body, using electric currents, microwaves, or ultrasound.

hydrotherapy The therapeutic use of water on the outside of the body, including the use of exercise pools, whirlpools, and showers.

laser therapy The use of lasers to reduce pain, inflammation, and swelling.

traction A therapeutic procedure in which part of the body is placed under tension, as by the attachment of a weight.

ultrasound The use of sound waves to treat soft tissues.

patient's life. I also thought it would be better than being a physician, since the therapists were able to spend a significantly greater amount of time interacting with their patients."

Jenni's primary duty is treating patients with a variety of musculoskeletal conditions. "This involves evaluation of the patient's condition and development of a plan of treatment specific to that patient's needs," she explains. "Treatment may include manual therapy techniques, passive stretching techniques, therapeutic exercises, body mechanics and postural training, balance activities, and use of therapeutic modalities." As a therapist in an outpatient setting, Jenni sees 12 to 14 patients per day.

In addition to treating patients, Jenni is responsible for documenting all treatment, deciding how to charge patients for services rendered, and serving as the manager of her clinic. As manager, she is responsible for making sure the clinic is compliant with all federal and state laws regarding the delivery of physical therapy, hiring staff, making sure the clinic is operating on budget, and overseeing the staff at the center.

Jenni also promotes physical therapy to physicians and potential patients. "This may mean that I shadow a physician for part of a day," she says, "or participate in a health fair. Additionally, I give lectures to runners in the Chicago area who are training for marathons on various topics such as how to perform proper stretching or how to strengthen their core muscles."

To Be a Successful Physical Therapist, You Should . . .

- like working with people
- have strong communication skills
- be able to work independently and as part of a team
- be creative
- be in good physical condition

DO I HAVE WHAT IT TAKES TO BE A PHYSICAL THERAPIST?

Physical therapists are respected members of the team of health care professionals involved in a patient's treatment and rehabilitation. Because physical therapists work not only with patients but also with other health care professionals, good communication skills are essential to this career. It is also a plus to have a positive attitude and an outgoing personality. Physical therapists must also be committed to lifelong learning because new developments in technology and medicine mean that therapists must continually update their knowledge.

Physical therapy requires a great deal of creativity on the part of the therapist. No two patients are alike, and no two will respond the same way to the same treatment. The physical therapist must be aware of a patient's needs and condition and be flexible enough to adapt therapy specifically to the patient.

HOW DO I BECOME A PHYSICAL THERAPIST?

Education

Jenni earned a bachelor's degree in kinesiology (the study of human movement) from Indiana University in Bloomington, Indiana, and a master's degree in physical therapy from Washington University in St. Louis, Missouri. "Physical therapy [graduate] programs require a four-year undergraduate degree," she says, "which may be in the area of the applicant's choosing. However, all physical therapy schools require certain pre-requisites, although this can vary slightly from school to school. Most schools require two semesters of chemistry, two semesters of physics, one semester of statistics, one semester of anatomy, and one semester of physiology, psychology, and human development."

High School

Competition for entering master's degree physical therapy programs is intense, so you should begin planning your career while still in high school. Courses in mathematics, biology, chemistry, physics, and other sciences should be part of your curriculum. You should also work on developing strong communication skills by taking English, speech, and writing classes.

An interest in sports and physical education will give you more insight into the functions of the body. Social sciences and psychology courses will bring you greater understanding of people. A physical therapist works with many different people from a variety of cultures, and therapists should be sensitive to each individual's concerns.

Postsecondary Training

Physical therapists attain their professional skills through extensive education that takes place both in the classroom and in clinical settings. You should attend a school accredited by the Commission on Accreditation in Physical Therapy Education (CAPTE) to receive the most thorough education. CAPTE now only accredits schools offering postbaccalaureate degrees (master's and doctorate degrees), and you will need one of these degrees to practice physical therapy. Previously, CAPTE had accredited bachelor's degree programs; however, this change was made to give students an appropriate amount of time to study liberal arts as well as a physical therapy curriculum. Course work should include classes in the humanities as well as those geared for the profession, such as anatomy, human growth and development, and therapeutic procedures. Clinical experience is done as supervised fieldwork in such settings as hospitals, home care agencies, and nursing homes. According to the American Physical Therapy Association (APTA), there are 61 accredited programs offering master's degrees and 148 offering doctorates in physical therapy. Visit the APTA's Web site (http://www.apta.org) for a listing of accredited programs.

Seven Specialties of Physical Therapy

- *Cardiopulmonary physical therapy* is concerned with the heart and lungs.

- *Clinical electrophysiology physical therapy* is concerned with the effects of electrical stimulation on the body.

- *Geriatrics physical therapy* is concerned with treatment of the elderly.

- *Neurology physical therapy* is concerned with the nervous system.

- *Orthopedics physical therapy* is concerned with the skeleton.

- *Pediatrics physical therapy* is concerned with treatment of children.

- *Sports physical therapy* is concerned with athletics and exercise.

Certification or Licensing

Specialist certification of physical therapists, while not a requirement for employment, is a desirable advanced credential. The American Board of Physical Therapy Specialties (ABPTS), an appointed group of the American Physical Therapy Association, certifies physical therapists who demonstrate specialized knowledge and advanced clinical proficiency in a specialty area of physical therapy practice and who pass a certifying examination. The seven areas of specialization are cardiopulmonary, clinical electrophysiology, neurology, orthopaedics, pediatrics, geriatrics, and sports. Jenni is certified as an orthopedic clinical specialist.

Upon graduating from an accredited physical therapy educational program, all physical therapists must successfully complete a national examination. Other licensing requirements vary by state. You will need to check with the licensing board of the state in which you hope to work for specific information.

Internships and Volunteerships

Students in physical therapy programs must participate in clinical education, although the number and length of rotations varies by school. "During clinical rotations," Jenni says, "the student treats patients under the supervision of a clinical instructor who is a practicing licensed physical therapist. My school required five clinical rotations. One rotation had to take place in an acute care setting, one in an outpatient setting, and one in a rehab hospital setting. The final two could be in pediatrics, home health, or another specialty area."

Volunteer work at local hospitals, health clinics, retirement homes, and other places that involve contact with both health care professionals and their patients will also help prepare you for this career.

WHO WILL HIRE ME?

Approximately 155,000 physical therapists are employed in the United States. Physical therapy offers a broad range of employment opportunities. About 60 percent of physical therapists work in hospitals and in offices of physical therapists. Others work in rehabilitation centers, health care clinics, physical therapy centers, community health centers, nursing homes, homes, hospices, schools, pediatric centers, sports facilities, and research institutions. Many companies in manufacturing and other areas employ physical therapists in corporate and industrial physical therapy departments.

WHERE CAN I GO FROM HERE?

In a hospital or other health care facility, one may rise from being a staff physical therapist to being the chief physical therapist and then director of the department. Administrative responsibilities are usually given to those physical therapists who have had several years of experience plus the personal qualities that prepare them for undertaking this kind of assignment.

After serving in a hospital or other institution for several years, some physical therapists open their own practices or go into a group practice, both of which often pay higher salaries. Jenni says she would like to either open her own physical therapy practice or teach at a physical therapy program while continuing to treat patients on a part-time basis.

WHAT ARE THE SALARY RANGES?

Salaries for physical therapists depend on experience and type of employer. Physical therapists earned an annual average salary of $61,560 in 2004, according to the U.S. Department of Labor. According to a 2005 APTA member survey, most physical therapists (55.7 percent) earned between $45,001 and $70,000 annually. Slightly less than 1 percent of APTA members earned $25,000 or less, and slightly more than 3 percent earned $150,000 or more annually.

WHAT IS THE JOB OUTLOOK?

Employment of physical therapists is expected to grow much faster than the average, according to the *Occupational Outlook Handbook.* This positive may be tempered by federal legislation that imposes limits on reimbursement for therapy services.

Over the long run, the demand for physical therapists should continue to rise as a result of growth in the number of individuals with disabilities or limited function requiring therapy services, such as the elderly population. As the baby boom generation enters the prime age for heart attacks and strokes, there will be increasing demand for cardiac and physical rehabilitation. Future medical developments may also increase the survival rates of trauma victims who will need rehabilitative services. In addition, a growing number of employers are using physical therapists to evaluate worksites, develop exercise programs, and teach safe work habits to employees in the hope of reducing injuries.

Physicians

SUMMARY

Definition
Physicians diagnose, prescribe medicines for, and otherwise treat diseases and disorders of the human body. A physician may also perform surgery and often specializes in one aspect of medical care and treatment. Physicians hold either a doctor of medicine (M.D.) or osteopathic medicine (D.O.) degree.

Alternative Job Titles
Doctors

Salary Range
$42,700 to $160,000 to $240,000+

Educational Requirements
Bachelor's degree, medical degree (M.D. or D.O.), residency training

Certification or Licensing
Required by all states

Outlook
Faster than the average

High School Subjects
Anatomy and physiology
Biology
Chemistry
Health

Personal Interests
Helping people: physical health/medicine
Psychology
Science

If you have a strong interest in science and anatomy and physiology, care deeply about helping others, and are a strong academic achiever, then a career as a physician may be just right for you. Read on to learn more about the exciting work of physicians.

WHAT DOES A PHYSICIAN DO?

The greatest number of physicians are in private practice. They see patients by appointment in their offices and examining rooms, and visit patients who are confined to the hospital. In the hospital, they may perform operations or give other kinds of medical treatment. Some physicians also make calls on patients at home if the patient is not able to get to the physician's office or if the illness is an emergency.

Family physicians see patients of all ages and both sexes and will diagnose and treat those ailments that are not severe enough or unusual enough to require the services of a specialist. When special problems arise, however, the family physician will refer the patient to a specialist.

Not all physicians are engaged in private practice. Some are in academic medicine and teach in medical schools or teaching hospitals. Some are engaged only in research. Some are salaried employees of health maintenance organizations or other prepaid health care plans. Some are salaried hospital employees.

Some physicians, often called *medical officers,* are employed by the federal government, in such positions as public health, or in the service of the Department of Veterans Affairs. State and local governments also employ physicians for public health agency work. A large number of physicians serve with the armed forces, both in this country and overseas.

Large industrial firms employ *industrial physicians* or *occupational physicians* for two main reasons: to prevent illnesses that may be caused by certain kinds of work and to treat accidents or illnesses of employees. Although most industrial physicians are family physicians because of the wide variety of illnesses that they must recognize and treat, their knowledge must also extend to public health techniques and to understanding such relatively new hazards as radiation and the toxic effects of various chemicals, including insecticides.

A specialized type of industrial or occupational physician is the *flight surgeon.* Flight surgeons study the effects of high-altitude flying on the physical condition of flight personnel. They place members of the flight staff in special low-pressure and refrigeration chambers that simulate high-altitude conditions and study the reactions on their blood pressure, pulse and respiration rate, and body temperature.

Another growing specialty is the field of nuclear medicine. Some large hospitals have a nuclear research laboratory, which functions under the direction of a *chief of nuclear medicine,* who coordinates the activities of the lab with other hospital departments and medical personnel. These physicians perform tests using nuclear isotopes and use techniques that let physicians see and understand organs deep within the body.

M.D.s may become specialists in any of the 40 different medical care specialties. Many of these specialties are discussed in the "What Do I Need to Know About Health Care?" section of this book.

Doctors of osteopathic medicine (D.O.s), more commonly referred to as

---

Lingo to Learn

electrocardiogram (EKG) A visible record of the electrical activity occurring as the heart beats.

health maintenance organization (HMO) A network of doctors that provides comprehensive health care but limits the subscriber to referrals for care by outside specialists.

managed care A philosophy of health care that tries to keep medical costs down through education and preventive medicine.

otoscope A viewing instrument used to examine the outer ear canal and the eardrum.

outpatient Patient treated at the hospital but not admitted for extended care.

osteopaths, practice a medical discipline that uses refined and sophisticated manipulative therapy based on the late 19th century teachings of American Dr. Andrew Taylor Still. It embraces the idea of "whole person" medicine and looks upon the system of muscles, bones, and joints—particularly the spine—as reflecting the body's diseases and as being partially responsible for initiating disease processes. Osteopaths are medical doctors with additional specialized training in this unique approach. They practice in a wide range of fields, from environmental medicine, geriatrics, and nutrition to sports medicine and neurology, among others.

WHAT IS IT LIKE TO BE A PHYSICIAN?

Dr. Mark Jacobson has operated a solo practice in allergy, asthma, and immunology since 1996. His office is located in Hinsdale, Illinois. "I started out in internal medicine," he recalls. "I did not like the idea of only seeing older patients. I also did not like the idea of only seeing children and infants. For a while I considered family medicine, but I thought it would be too hard to know EVERYTHING about EVERYONE. I thought I would be more comfortable being an expert about a more limited area of medicine. I also liked the fact that in allergy the patients tend to get better and that there is a lot of opportunity for patient education—which is an aspect that I enjoy greatly."

When Mark arrives at his office each day, he responds to urgent phone calls and e-mails, and then he begins to see patients. "I spend about 40 minutes with each new patient and 15 to 20 minutes with each follow-up patient. While I am in the room with the patient, I am also writing down what they are telling me as well as what my plan is to do for them. It is pretty much a constant flow of seeing patients one after another. Occasionally, I must take a phone call from another doctor or from a patient who has an urgent question."

At the end of the day, Mark returns any phone calls that came in during the day. He also dictates a report for each of the patients referred to him by another physician (which is most of the time). "If I have any down time at all," he says, "I try to catch up on my reading. Some of this is reading medical journals, and some of it can now be done online. If my office hours end at 4:00 P.M, I am usually there until 5:00. On Tuesdays and Thursdays, I start after 12:00 and see patients until 7:00. I then stay later doing paperwork (sometimes as late as 10:00 or 11:00 P.M.) I do not work at all on Friday, Saturday, or Sunday, although my pager is always on since I am in solo practice."

Asked about the pros and cons of his job, Mark says that he enjoys working in the field of allergy/immunology because the patients actually tend to get better. "This is very gratifying and may be different than what is experienced in some of the other medical specialties," he says. He also enjoys interacting with patients of all ages, as well as the benefits of working as a sole practitioner. "Being a solo practitioner," he says, "I have lots of autonomy. I can set my own hours and spend as much time as each of my patients require." Mark says that one drawback to his specialty is that allergists do not spend much time seeing patients in hospital settings. "This may be good as far as making the day more predictable," he explains, "however, it means that we have less opportunity to mingle with our other medical colleagues."

Dr. Rick Kellerman is a family physician in Wichita, Kansas, and professor and chair of the Department of Family and Community Medicine at the University of Kansas School of Medicine-Wichita. In addition, he is the president-elect of the American Academy of Family Physicians. "A career in medicine offers the opportunity to make a difference in people's lives," he says. "I think I always knew that I wanted to be a physician," he

says. "My concept of being a physician was always that of a family physician. I was influenced by my family physicians growing up. They took an interest in me, my family, and were active in the community. During medical school, when I was assigned different specialty rotations, I always thought 'this is interesting, but I like the other disciplines also . . . and do I want to do just this one narrow specialty for the rest of my life?'"

The offices and examining rooms of most physicians are well equipped, attractive, well lighted, and well ventilated. There is usually at least one nurse-receptionist on the physician's staff, and there may be several nurses, a laboratory technician, one or more secretaries, a bookkeeper, or receptionist.

Physicians usually see patients by appointments that are scheduled according to individual requirements. They may reserve all mornings for hospital visits and surgery. They may see patients in the office only on certain days of the week.

Physicians in private practice have the advantages of working independently, but almost one-third of all physicians worked an average of 60 hours or more per week in 2002. Also, they may be called from their homes or offices in times of emergency. Telephone calls may come at any hour of the day or night. It is difficult for physicians to plan leisure-time activities because their plans may change without notice. One of the advantages of group practice is that members of the group rotate emergency duty.

The areas in most need of physicians are rural hospitals and medical centers.

More Lingo to Learn

preferred provider organization (PPO) A network of medical professionals that are under contract with insurance companies to provide care to individual subscribers.

preventive care A type of medical care that stresses the prevention of disease by teaching patients better eating habits and other healthy lifestyle choices.

residency A period of advanced medical training and education that normally follows graduation from medical school.

stethoscope An instrument used for listening to sounds within the body, primarily in the heart and lungs.

To Be a Successful Physician, You Should . . .

- be committed to helping people
- be compassionate and understanding
- have the stamina to work long and irregular hours
- have good communication skills
- inspire confidence and trust

Because the physician is normally working alone and covering a broad territory, the workday can be quite long, with little opportunity for vacation. Because placement in rural communities has become so difficult, some towns are providing scholarship money to students who pledge to work in the community for a number of years.

Physicians in academic medicine or in research have regular hours, work under good physical conditions, and often determine their own workload. Teaching and research physicians alike are usually provided with the best and most modern equipment.

DO I HAVE WHAT IT TAKES TO BE A PHYSICIAN?

If you work directly with patients, you need to have great sensitivity to their needs. Dr. Jacobson offers the following advice to future physicians: "treat your patients the way you yourself would want to be treated or the way you would want a loved one to be treated, such as your own grandmother. I have seen many physicians be rude to their patients, especially some of their older patients." Interpersonal skills are important, even in isolated research laboratories, since you must work and communicate with other scientists. Since new technology and discoveries happen at such a rapid rate, you must continually pursue further education to keep up with new treatments, tools, and medicines.

In addition to good interpersonal skills, physicians need a great deal of stamina to keep up with the many demands their jobs require. Physicians work long, irregular hours, including instances when they may be called from their homes or offices to attend to emergencies. Dedication is also necessary to keep up with the rigorous educational demands. "Physicians," says Dr. William Anderson, an allergy-immunology specialist at the Asthma & Allergy Center of Whatcom County, Bellingham, Washington, "must also live with and understand delayed gratification, spending years in school, followed by years in training as their peers pursuing non-medical careers are working and earning a living and 'climbing the corporate ladder.'"

For many physicians, the career's rewards far outweigh its demands. Helping sick people become well is both gratifying and uplifting. "I enjoy working with my patients, using my knowledge, expertise, and experience in improving the lives of my patients," Dr. Anderson says.

HOW DO I BECOME A PHYSICIAN?

Education

High School

High school students who plan to become physicians need to take a basic college preparatory curriculum, including English, history, social studies, math, and foreign languages.

Specific high school classes that will be helpful to prospective physicians include biology, chemistry, physics, and physiology. English and speech classes are also useful because doctors need to develop good communication skills, both written and oral.

Dr. Anderson offers the following advice to high school students interested in medical careers: "I would advise high school students to do their best in science and math classes to ensure that they enjoy such work. It would also be helpful to actually spend time with a physician to get an idea first-hand what it may be like to be a doctor, and to hear about how to become one. Interested students also should realize that it takes a lot of work, not only before becoming a doctor, but even afterwards. In private practice, a significant part of the work is directed toward ensuring that financial goals are achieved, and this requires a different knowledge base, that of the business side of medicine. Assistance and guidance in this area is available from professional associations. Financial success may require time and effort above what one may expect for this profession, and therefore, it must be an individual's desire in learning about med-

icine and the science of the human body, and the privilege to help others in a way no other profession can, that drives their passion to work as a physician."

Dr. Jacobson advises high school students interested in the field to enter the career "because you want to help other people and you are committed to lifelong learning. Do not go into it for the money; there are much easier ways to make a lot of money. Do not go into medicine because you think it is 'glamorous.' Most physician practices are not like *ER*, *Grey's Anatomy*, or *General Hospital*."

Postsecondary Training

In college, you should enroll in a program with a strong emphasis on the sciences,

---

Important Qualities for Med Students

Dr. Rick Kellerman, a family physician in Wichita, Kansas, and professor and chair of the Department of Family and Community Medicine at the University of Kansas School of Medicine-Wichita, lists the following personal and professional qualities as being the most important for medical students.

- native intelligence
- strong motivation
- caring personality
- ability to communicate (verbal and writing skills)
- integrity
- desire to serve

such as a premed program. You can also follow a liberal arts program and major in biology or chemistry. In general, students take classes in physics, biology, mathematics, inorganic and organic chemistry, as well as classes in the humanities and social sciences.

During the junior or senior year of college, students should arrange to take the Medical College Admission Test (MCAT). This test, which is given twice a year, evaluates students' ability in four areas: verbal facility, quantitative ability, knowledge of the humanities and social sciences, and knowledge of biology, chemistry, and physics.

Medical schools are highly competitive. In addition to MCAT scores, applicants must submit transcripts and letters of recommendation. In addition to academics, an applicant's character, personality, leadership qualities, and participation in extracurricular activities are also taken into account.

During the first two years of medical school, students spend most of their time in the laboratory or the classroom. They take courses such as anatomy, physiology, pharmacology, psychology, microbiology, pathology, medical ethics, and medical law. They also learn how to take medical histories, examine patients, and recognize basic symptoms.

The last two years are spent working with patients in hospitals and clinics, under the supervision of practicing physicians. Students spend set periods of time, called "rotations," in internal medicine, family medicine, obstetrics and gynecology, pediatrics, psychiatry, and surgery.

While remaining closely supervised, the medical student is actively involved in patient treatment as part of a hospital medical team. The student also continues to do course work. In addition to the clinical sciences, there may be work in business areas, such as decision analysis and cost containment.

Upon completion of medical school, students receive either the doctor of medicine (M.D.) or the doctor of osteopathic medicine (D.O.) degree and continue their training through medical residencies. Residents are actively involved in patient treatment as part of a hospital medical team. The residency for a family physician usually lasts three years and involves long hours of demanding work and intensive study.

Dr. Jacobson advises students to "keep in mind that there are many different specialties, and each will offer you a different kind of lifestyle, and I am not talking about the money. Keep in mind how much time you would like to spend with your family. Do you want a specialty that is primarily outpatient such as allergy, or more inpatient such as surgery or emergency medicine? Do you like handling a lot of emergencies or do you prefer for things to be more predictable? For those who want to be a physician, but are not comfortable with patient contact, you can pick a specialty such as radiology or pathology."

Physicians must continue to learn throughout their careers in order to stay up-to- date with current medical developments. "Medical education doesn't stop at medical school or residency," says

Dr. Kellerman. "Physicians have continuing medical education that is ongoing throughout their careers. So if you don't have good study skills, this may not be the career for you. It is a requirement that you stay up-to-date in medicine!"

Certification or Licensing

Board certification is available in many medical specialties. This credential, though voluntary, signifies that the physician is highly qualified in his or her particular specialty.

At an early point in the residency period, all physicians, both M.D.s and D.O.s., must pass a state medical board examination in order to obtain a license and enter practice. Each state sets its own requirements and issues its own licenses, although some states will accept licenses from other states. Physicians seeking licensure must graduate from an accredited medical school, complete residency postgraduate training, and pass a licensing examination administered by their state's board of medical examiners. Some states have reciprocity agreements so that a physician licensed to practice in one state may be automatically licensed in another state without having to pass another examination.

Internships and Volunteerships

After receiving their medical degrees, nearly all M.D.s continue their training through medical residencies—paid on-the-job training in a hospital in the physician's chosen specialty. Doctors of osteopathic medicine usually take part in a 12-month rotating internship after they

FYI

Most people in the United States can expect to live well into their 70s. In 1850, however, the average life span was only about 40 years. Lengthened life span is largely the result of centuries of medical advances.

graduate, and then enter a medical residency to receive more training.

Volunteer opportunities are available in local hospitals or other health care facilities. You can gain exposure to a medical environment and experience helping people, even if your job involves delivering flowers or filling water pitchers in patients' rooms. You can also benefit from simply talking to physicians about their work.

WHO WILL HIRE ME?

After physicians complete their residency programs, they are ready to enter practice. They may choose to open a solo private practice, join a partnership or group practice, or take a salaried job in a clinic or managed care (HMO or PPO) network. Salaried positions are also available with federal and state agencies, neighborhood health centers, and the military, including the Department of Veterans Affairs.

Many new physicians choose to join existing practices instead of attempting to start their own. Establishing a new practice is costly, and it may take time to build a patient base. In a clinic, group practice, or partnership, physicians share the costs for medical equipment and staff salaries, and are able to establish a wider patient base.

Physicians who hope to join an existing practice may find leads through their medical school or residency. During these experiences, they work with many members of the medical community, some of who may be able to recommend them to appropriate practices.

Another approach would be to check the various medical professional journals, which often run ads for physician positions. Aspiring physicians can also hire a medical placement agency to assist them in the job search.

Physicians who hope to work for a managed care organization or government sponsored clinic should contact the source directly for information on position availability and application procedures.

The majority of physicians practice in urban areas, near hospitals and educational centers. Therefore, competition for patients is likely to be higher in these areas. In contrast, rural communities and small towns are often in need of doctors and may be promising places for young physicians to establish practices.

WHERE CAN I GO FROM HERE?

Physicians who work in a managed-care setting or for a large group or corporation can advance by opening a private practice. The average physician in private practice does not advance in the

accustomed sense of the word. Their progress consists of advancing in skill and understanding, in numbers of patients, and in income. They may be made a fellow in a professional specialty or elected to an important office in the American Medical Association or American Osteopathic Association. Teaching and research positions may also increase a physician's status.

Some physicians may become directors of a laboratory, managed-care facility, hospital department, or medical school program. Some may move into hospital administration positions.

Physicians can achieve recognition by conducting research in new medicines, treatments, and cures, and publishing their findings in medical journals. Participation in professional organizations can also bring prestige.

A physician can advance by pursuing further education in a subspecialty or a second field such as biochemistry or microbiology.

Dr. Kellerman enjoys his current career, but says that he is unsure if he will remain in the same position in 5 or 10 years. "An advantage of family medicine

FYI

The ancient Greek physician Hippocrates is credited with the belief that disease has physical, not magical, causes.

is the variety of things I can do," he says. "I've been a rural solo physician, run a residency program, worked in an inner-city clinic, and now chair an academic department. I've never worried much about being employed in family medicine because I can fit into so many positions."

"I see myself in the future doing the same work that I am doing presently," Dr. Anderson predicts. I am fortunate to be able to care for both children and adults as a specialist. I hope to spend more time educating groups, both patients and primary care physicians in the field of allergy/immunology. I will probably scale back a bit and spend more time on my recreational pursuits."

In 5 or 10 years, Dr. Jacobson hopes to still be in private practice, "although," he says, "I hope to have at least one additional associate within the next couple of years."

WHAT ARE THE SALARY RANGES?

Physicians have among the highest average earnings of any occupational group. The level of income for any individual physician depends on a number of factors, such as region of the country, economic status of the patients, and the physician's specialty, skill, experience, professional reputation, and personality. Income tends to vary less across geographic regions, however, than across specialties. The median income for all physicians is $160,000 per year, according to the American Medical Association.

Most physicians earn between $120,000 and $240,00 annually. According to the U.S. Department of Labor, the mean income in 2004 for family physicians was $137,980; general surgeons, $181,850; anesthesiologists, $174,610; obstetricians/gynecologists, $180,660; and pediatricians, $140,000.

In 2005-2006, the average first-year resident received a stipend of about $42,070 a year, according to the Association of American Medical Colleges, depending on the type of residency, the size of the hospital, and the geographic area. Sixth-year residents earned about $51,284 a year. If the physician enters private practice, earnings during the first year may not be impressive. As the patients increase in number, however, earnings will also increase.

Physicians who complete their residencies but have no other experience begin work with the Department of Veterans Affairs at salaries of about $44,400, in addition to other cash benefits of up to $13,000.

Related Jobs

- dentists
- health care managers
- holistic physicians
- nurse practitioners
- optometrists
- oral and maxillofacial surgeons
- physician assistants

Salaried doctors usually earn fringe benefits such as health and dental insurance, paid vacations, and the opportunity to participate in retirement plans. Physicians who are self-employed must provide their own insurance coverage. Those who are employed by a clinic or managed-care organization usually receive a benefits package that includes insurance and paid time off.

WHAT IS THE JOB OUTLOOK?

Employment of physicians is expected to grow faster than the average for all occupations through the next decade, according to the U.S. Department of Labor. "I would tell young adults," says Dr. Anderson, "that the world will always need good physicians, and that if one has a burning desire to understand human biology (physiology) and would like to use their knowledge to improve the quality of life of others, then medicine may be a good career. Students should understand that although there is delayed gratification when it comes to "getting a real job" in medicine, that is, the opportunity to work independently and receive a salary, there can be fun and excitement in the training process, as well as the instant gratification that comes with helping others through times of trouble."

One reason for the strong employment demand is population growth. People are living longer, requiring more health care as they age. Another reason for the growth is the availability of better health care. Physicians can perform more tests and treat conditions that were once untreatable. In addition, the widespread use of medical insurance plans help to make expensive procedures more affordable to patients.

More physicians will also be needed for medical research, public health, rehabilitation, and industrial medicine. New technology will allow physicians to perform more procedures to treat ailments once thought incurable.

Because most physicians choose to practice in urban areas, these areas are often oversupplied and fiercely competitive. Physicians just entering the field may find it difficult to enter a practice and build a patient base in a big city. There is a growing need, however, for physicians in rural communities and small towns. Physicians who are willing to relocate to these areas should have excellent job prospects.

SECTION 3

Do It Yourself

If you've made it this far through the book, it's probably because a career in health care is starting to sound like a definite possibility. Whether you're interested in caring for patients, writing about medical issues, repairing or operating medical equipment, or some other area, the career possibilities in health care are endless! While you won't be able to work as a nurse, doctor, or other health care professional until you receive training in college, there are many things you can do now to experience this field. Here are some suggestions and activities to explore this fast-growing industry. Read on and be inspired to make your dream into reality—STAT!

❑ READ, READ, AND READ!

The best way to investigate this industry is by reading about it. Start with your school library or guidance office to find all career books and articles on different health care careers. Browse the periodical section of your local library and read what the professionals read, such as the *Journal of the American Medical Association, NurseWeek,* and the *Journal of the American Physical Therapy Association.* Check the Internet as well, since many magazines also offer online versions of their issues. Some articles may be interesting, others over your head, but at the very least you'll get a feel for the industry and its lingo. Magazines and industry periodicals also list available employment opportunities—this is a great way to learn about the different job markets throughout the nation. For a great list of books and periodicals about health care, check out the chapter "Read a Book" in Section 4.

❑ SURF THE WEB

The Internet is an excellent place to learn more about health care. You can find information on health care associations, discussion groups, competitions, educational programs, glossaries, company information, worker profiles and interviews, and the list goes on and on. So surf the Web, and begin learning about health care! Check out "Surf the Web" in Section 4.

❑ JOIN AN ASSOCIATION

Many health care professional associations offer membership to college students. Typical membership benefits include the opportunity to participate in association-sponsored competitions, seminars, and conferences; subscriptions to magazines (some of them geared specifically toward students—that provide the latest industry information); mentoring and networking opportunities; and access to financial aid. Some health care associations even offer membership to high school students and individuals who are simply interested in health care. The American Association of Critical-Care Nurses, for example, offers consumer membership to non-nurses who are interested in the field of critical care nursing. Visit "Look to the Pros" in Section 4 for more information on associations that offer student membership.

❏ USEFUL HIGH SCHOOL CLASSES

In addition to classes like anatomy and physiology, biology, chemistry, and mathematics, you should also consider taking less traditional courses. Did you know that many dental schools often require their students to take art classes to help improve their hand coordination and dexterity? Some art classes to consider are painting or sculpture. (Of course, if you want to become a medical illustrator, then art classes should already be at the top of your list!) Are you interested in working as a dietitian? Then enroll in home economics classes to learn different ways to prepare food and study nutrition. You get the idea.

In addition, if you plan to take a foreign language, you may want to opt for Latin over popular languages such as French or Spanish, since many medical terms are rooted in this ancient language. Also, don't forget to take classes that require plenty of researching and writing, as well as public speaking—such skills will prove helpful with charting and communicating with patients.

❏ VISIT MUSEUMS

What early tools did dentists use? Were George Washington's teeth really made of wood? Who is St. Apollonia? Visit the National Museum of Dentistry, located in Baltimore, Maryland, to learn the answers to these questions, and much more. The National Museum of Dentistry, affiliated with the Smithsonian Institution, has exhibits tracing the history of dentistry, its prominent contributors, and innovations for the future. Along with its permanent collection, the museum has special exhibits that travel to different museums throughout the nation. Visit http://www.dentalmuseum.umaryland.edu for more details.

If you are interested in the history of surgery, you'll want to visit the Museum of Surgical Science in Chicago, Illinois. Exhibits include medical artifacts such as early surgical tools, orthopedic pieces dating back to the Civil War era, and a working iron lung. The museum also presents new innovations and technology in surgical practice. Visit http://www.imss.org to learn more, or search the Web for traveling health-themed exhibits coming to your city.

❏ TAKE A FIRST AID CLASS

While you may still be too young to enroll, for example, in nursing school or an occupational therapy program, there are several courses available for your age group. The Red Cross offers first aid classes for all ages and instruction on techniques, such as CPR and the Heimlich maneuver, to use during medical emergencies. Visit http://www.redcross.org/services/hss/courses for available classes. Your park district or community center may also offer such courses. If your dream is to be a health care professional, a first aid certificate is your first step!

❏ ATTEND A SUMMER CAMP

Don't expect swimming activities and nightly bonfires. Instead, gear up to get "hands-on" experience in the medical field through class lectures, laboratory work, and basic medical procedures. You can search the Internet for health care-themed summer camps in your area. If you cannot locate one near your home, why not contact a local hospital about developing a program? Summer programs are covered in depth in Section 4: What Can I Do Right Now: Get Involved: A Directory of Camps, Programs, and Competitions. Visit the section for further information.

❑ TOUR A MEDICAL FACILITY

Many hospitals offer guided tours to give students a firsthand view of how patients receive medical care. Hospitals in the University Healthcare System of Augusta, Georgia, for example, offer general tours of the pediatric department and emergency department for elementary students, with a more detailed tour for high school students including visits to the radiology department and laboratory. For more information on this program, visit http://www.universityhealth.org/160.cfm.

Tour options are available throughout the United States. Contact the community relations department of your local hospital to learn more about available programs.

❑ VOLUNTEER, VOLUNTEER, VOLUNTEER!

In the past, hospital volunteers were called candy stripers, named for the red and white candy cane–like smocks they were required to wear. You won't have to wear this garb in most hospitals, but you'll get to work in various departments of the hospital, assist hospital staff, and earn valuable school service points. As part of the volunteer team, you may be given responsibilities such as assisting nurses with basic tasks, monitoring visitor passes, delivering mail and flowers to patients, assisting in the preoperative holding area, and escorting or running simple errands for patients. Expect to work at least 40 hours a year (depending on the needs of the facility), take a required tuberculosis test, and participate in a hospital orientation. Contact your local hospital to learn more about its volunteer program. Volunteer opportunities also exist at nursing homes—you can help with patient activities such as bingo, holiday parties, or help write letters for those suffering from arthritis or dementia. Health clinics also appreciate volunteers to help them with patient registration and general office work.

❑ TAKE ADVANTAGE OF THE HEALTH CAREERS OPPORTUNITY PROGRAM

The Health Careers Opportunity Program (HCOP) is a federally funded program that helps recruit and/or assist disadvantaged students interested in health care careers. Services are offered to students at the high school and college level who are disadvantaged financially, culturally, or by education.

Students at the junior high and high school level can take advantage of career field trips, occupation fairs, and career conferences sponsored by HCOP. One activity is the "Day With Health Professionals" presentation, where doctors, nurses, therapists, and other workers talk about their daily duties and responsibilities.

HCOP also offers various programs to motivate and prepare students for the next step: a health career after high school graduation. Activities include a health careers summer camp, a medical anatomy and physiology program, and a preparation program for technical careers such as occupational therapy assistant, medical laboratory technician, or biotechnology technician.

HCOP also has a mentorship program, which matches students with professionals already established in the medical field. Students are encouraged to meet with their mentors for inspiration, or to receive help with personal or educational challenges

Visit http://www.bhpr.hrsa.gov/diversity/hcop for more information, to locate a local HCOP program, or to download an application.

❏ GET A PART-TIME JOB

Jobs in the health care industry can take different forms—whether giving direct medical attention, organizing research and data, or providing the tools and equipment needed by medical professionals. Ultimately a job in health care means you want to help others! Part-time employment can be your test—do you have what

it takes? Doctor's offices, clinics, and nursing homes can be great sources of employment at the part-time level. You may be asked to answer phones, fill out health forms, or file paperwork and test results, billing, or patient registration. Neighborhood pharmacies also hire students to help keep inventory or work the register. It may not be glamorous work, but you'll be providing much-needed and valued assistance. Hospitals are another source of student employment. You may be hired to work in the dietary department to help provide meals to patients as approved by registered dietitians, or in the transport department to move patients to different testing areas within the hospital quickly and safely. Notify your school guidance counselor about your interest in a part-time job—they often have knowledge of such job openings. The employment section of your local newspaper is another great source when job searching.

❏ "SHADOW" A HEALTH CARE WORKER

Do you want to experience a day in the life of a pharmacist? Or pediatric nurse? Or phlebotomist? Job shadowing is the perfect way to get a feel for their routine and the responsibilities of these and other health care careers. Community Hospital in Munster, Indiana, for example, offers a job-shadowing program for those interested in the field of nursing. After orientation, students are teamed with nurses of various specialties. Students are able to "work" alongside nurses as they treat patients in cardiac rehab, triage in the emergency department, and give various treatments to patients. Talk to your guidance counselor to learn more about job-shadowing programs available in your area.

Do you have relatives who work in the health care industry? Inquire if their places of employment participate in the annual Take Your Daughter/Son To Work Day. This popular program designates a day to encourage children to see what their parents do while at work. Lectures and special activities and games are planned to make the day entertaining as well as educational. Visit http://www.daughtersandsonstowork.org for more information.

Consider the following points before participating in a shadow program. You will be a representative of the hospital, clinic, or business, even if it's just for a day. Make sure you conduct yourself in a professional and courteous manner, especially when interacting with patients or customers. Dress appropriately—no jeans, cutoffs, or other pieces of apparel or jewelry deemed sloppy.

For more information on job shadowing, visit http://www.jobshadow.org.

❏ PLAN A HEALTH FAIR

Does your school or community sponsor a health fair? If not, organize one! Health fairs provide a venue for health care providers, businesses, and associations to promote their services. You can ask your local Red Cross chapter to give first aid classes, local doctors to provide high blood pressure screenings, even pediatric dentists to show children the right way to brush and floss teeth. The possibilities are endless. If the thought of putting on such a show is daunting, then start small. Why not present a "germ show" aimed at the pre-school level? Talk about the types of germs—helpful and harmful; use puppets to show kids the proper way to wash their hands, and the consequences of passing on germs to others. You will be teaching kids how to help keep themselves healthy, as well be on the right track to a new career: public health educator!

SECTION 4

WHAT CAN I DO RIGHT NOW?

Get Involved: A Directory of Camps, Programs, and Competitions

Now that you've read about some of the different careers available in health care, you may be anxious to experience this line of work for yourself, to find out what it's really like. Or, perhaps you already feel certain that this is the career path for you and want to get started on it right away. Whichever is the case, this section is for you! There are plenty of things you can do right now to learn about health care careers while gaining valuable experience. Just as important, you'll get to meet new friends and see new places, too.

In the following pages you will find programs designed to pique your interest in health care and start preparing you for a career. You already know that this field is complex, and that to work in it you need a solid education. Since the first step toward an health care career will be gaining that education, we've found 40 programs that will start you on your way. Some are special introductory sessions, others are actual college courses—one of them may be right for you. Take time to read the listings and see how each compares to your situation: how committed you are to health care, how much of your money and free time you're willing to devote to it, and how the program will help you after high school. These listings are divided into categories, with the type of program printed right after its name or the name of the sponsoring organization.

❑ THE CATEGORIES
Camps
When you see an activity that is classified as a camp, don't automatically start packing your tent and mosquito repellent. Where academic study is involved, the term "camp" often simply means a residential program including both educational and recreational activities. It's sometimes hard to differentiate between such camps and other study programs, but if the sponsoring organization calls it a camp, so do we! For an extended list of camps, visit http://www.kidscamps.com.

College Courses/Summer Study
These terms are linked because most college courses offered to students your age must take place in the summer, when you are out of school. At the same time, many colleges and universities that want to attract future students and give them a head start in higher education sponsor summer study programs. Summer study of almost any type is a good idea because it keeps your mind and your study skills sharp over the long vacation. Summer study at a college offers any number of additional benefits, including giving you the tools to make a well-informed decision about your future academic career. Study options, including some impressive college and university programs, account

for most of the listings in this section—primarily because higher education is so crucial to every health care career.

Competitions

Competitions are fairly self-explanatory, but you should know that there are only a few in this book because many health care-related competitions are at the local and regional levels and so again are impractical to list here. What this means, however, is that if you are interested in entering a competition, you shouldn't have much trouble finding one yourself. Your guidance counselor or science or health teachers can help you start searching in your area.

Employment and Internship Opportunities

As you may already know from experience, employment opportunities for teenagers can be very limited. This is particularly true for most careers in health care, although you might consider working in the food service or records department of your local hospital to at least gain exposure to career opportunities in health care. Even internships are most often reserved for college students who have completed at least one or two years of study in the field. Still, if you're very determined to find an internship or paid position in health care, there may be ways to find one. See the "Do It Yourself" section in this book for some suggestions.

Field Experience

This is something of a catchall category for activities that don't exactly fit the other descriptions. But anything called a field experience in this book is always a good opportunity to get out and explore the work of health care professionals.

Membership

When an organization is in this category, it simply means that you are welcome to pay your dues and become a card-carrying member. Formally joining any organization brings the benefits of meeting others who share your interests, finding opportunities to get involved, and keeping up with current events. Depending on how active you are, the contacts you make and the experiences you gain may help when the time comes to apply to colleges or look for a job.

In some organizations, you pay a special student rate and receive benefits similar to regular members. Many organizations, however, are now starting student branches with their own benefits and publications. As in any field, make sure you understand exactly what the benefits of membership are before you join.

Finally, don't let membership dues discourage you from making contact with these organizations. Some charge dues as low as $25 because they know that students are perpetually short of funds. When the annual dues are higher, think of the money as an investment in your future and then consider if it is too much to pay.

❏ PROGRAM DESCRIPTIONS

Once you've started to look at the individual listings themselves, you'll find that they contain a lot of information. Naturally, there is a general description of each program, but wherever possible we also have included the following details.

Application Information

Each listing notes how far in advance you'll need to apply for the program or position, but the simple rule is to apply as far in advance as possible. This ensures that you won't miss out on a great opportunity simply because other people got there ahead of you. It also means that you will get a timely decision on your application, so if you are not accepted, you'll still have some time to apply elsewhere. As for the things that make up your application—essays, recommendations, etc.—we've tried to cover what's involved, but be sure to contact the program about specific requirements before you submit anything.

Background Information

This includes such information as the date the program was established, the name of the organization that is sponsoring it financially, and the faculty and staff who will be there for you. This can help you—and your family—gauge the quality and reliability of the program.

Classes and Activities

Classes and activities change from year to year, depending on popularity, availability of instructors, and many other factors. Nevertheless, colleges and universities quite consistently offer the same or similar classes, even in their summer sessions. Courses like "Introduction to Nursing" and "Biology 101," for example, are simply indispensable. So you can look through the listings and see which programs offer foundational courses like these and which offer courses on more variable topics. As for activities, we note when you have access to recreational facilities on campus, and it's usually a given that special social and cultural activities will be arranged for most programs.

Contact Information

Wherever possible, we have given the title of the person whom you should contact instead of the name because people change jobs so frequently. If no title is given and you are telephoning an organization, simply tell the person who answers the phone the name of the program that interests you and he or she will forward your call. If you are writing, include the line "Attention: Summer Study Program" (or whatever is appropriate after "Attention") somewhere on the envelope. This will help to ensure that your letter goes to the person in charge of that program.

Credit

Where academic programs are concerned, we sometimes note that high school or college credit is available to those who have completed them. This means that the program can count toward your high school diploma or a future college degree just like a regular course. Obviously, this can be very useful, but it's important to note that rules about accepting such credit vary from school to school. Before you commit to a program offering high school credit, check with your guidance counselor to see if it is acceptable to your school. As for programs offering college credit, check with your chosen college (if you have one) to see if they will accept it.

Eligibility and Qualifications

The main eligibility requirement to be concerned about is age or grade in school. A term frequently used in relation to grade level is "rising," as in "rising senior": someone who will be a senior when the next school year begins. This is especially important where summer programs are concerned. A number of university-based programs make admissions decisions partly in consideration of GPA, class rank, and standardized test scores. This is mentioned in the listings, but you must contact the program for specific numbers. If you are worried that your GPA or your ACT scores, for example, aren't good enough, don't let them stop you from applying to programs that consider such things in the admissions process. Often, a fine essay or even an example of your dedication and eagerness can compensate for statistical weaknesses.

Facilities

We tell you where you'll be living, studying, eating, and having fun during these programs, but there isn't enough room to go into all the details. Some of those details can be important: what is and isn't accessible for people with disabilities, whether the site of a summer program has air-conditioning, and how modern the laboratory and computer equipment are. You can expect most program brochures and application materials to address these concerns, but if you still have questions about the facilities, just call the program's administration and ask.

Financial Details

While a few of the programs listed here are fully underwritten by collegiate and corporate sponsors, most of them rely on you for at least some of their funding. The 2006 prices and fees are given here, but you should bear in mind that costs rise slightly almost every year. You and your parents must take costs into consideration when choosing a program. We always try to note where financial aid is available, but really, most programs will do their best to ensure that a shortage of funds does not prevent you from taking part.

Residential vs. Commuter Options

Simply put, some programs prefer that participating students live with other participants and staff members, others do not, and still others leave the decision entirely to the students themselves. As a rule, residential programs are suitable for young people who live out of town or even out of state, as well as for local residents. They generally provide a better overview of college life than programs in which you're only on campus for a few hours a day, and they're a way to test how well you cope with living away from home. Commuter programs may be viable only if you live near the program site or if you can stay with relatives who do. Bear in mind that for residential programs especially, the travel between your home and the location of the activity is almost always your responsibility and can significantly increase the cost of participation.

❏ FINALLY . . .

Ultimately, there are three important things to bear in mind concerning all of the programs listed in this volume. The first is that things change. Staff members come and go, funding is added or withdrawn, supply and demand determine which programs continue and which terminate. Dates, times, and costs vary widely due to a number of factors. Because of this, the information we give you, although as current and detailed as possible, is just not enough on which to base your final decision. If you are interested in a program, you simply must write, call, fax, or e-mail the organization concerned to get the latest and most complete information available. This has the added benefit of putting you in touch with someone who can deal with your individual questions and problems.

Another important point to keep in mind when considering these programs is that the people who run them provided the information printed here. The editors of this book haven't attended the programs and don't endorse them: we simply give you the information with which to begin your own research. And after all, we can't pass judgment because you're the only one who can decide which programs are right for you.

The final thing to bear in mind is that the programs listed here are just the tip of the iceberg. No book can possibly cover all of the opportunities that are available to you—partly because they are so numerous and are constantly coming and going, and partly because some are waiting to be discovered. For instance, you may be very interested in taking a college course but don't see the college that interests you in the listings. Call their admissions office! Even if they don't have a special program for high school students, they might be able to make some kind of arrangements for you to visit or sit in on a class. Use the ideas behind these listings and take the initiative to turn them into opportunities!

❏ THE PROGRAMS

Academic Study Associates (ASA)
College Courses/Summer Study

Academic Study Associates has been offering residential and commuter pre-college summer programs for young people for more than 20 years. It offers college credit classes and enrichment opportunities in a variety of academic fields, including natural sciences (which includes chemistry, mathematics, psychology, and science—important classes for future health care professionals), at the University of Massachusetts-Amherst and the University of California-Berkeley, as well as institutions abroad. In addition to classroom work, students participate in field trips, mini-clinics, and extracurricular activities. Programs are usually three to four weeks in length. Fees and deadlines vary for these programs—visit the ASA Web site for further details. Options are also available for middle school students.

Academic Study Associates (ASA)

ASA Programs
375 West Broadway, Suite 200
New York, NY 10012-4324
800-752-2250
summer@asaprograms.com
http://www.asaprograms.com/home/
asa_home.asp

American Assembly for Men in Nursing

Membership

The assembly is a support organization for male nurses. Members of the general public who have an interest in nursing can apply to become associate members. Contact the assembly for more information.

American Assembly for Men in Nursing Foundation

PO Box 130220
Birmingham, AL 35213-0220
205-802-7551
aamn@aamn.org
http://www.aamn.org

American Association of Critical-Care Nurses (AACN)

Membership

This is a professional association for critical-care nurses. Members of the public who are interested in the field of critical-care nursing can apply for affiliate membership. Members receive access to literature databases at the AACN Web site; subscriptions to *Critical Care Nurse, American Journal of Critical Care, AACN News,* and AACN's e-newsletter *Critical Care Newsline;* and are eligible for schol-arships, grants, and awards. Contact the association for more information.

American Association of Critical-Care Nurses

101 Columbia
Aliso Viejo, CA 92656-4109
800-899-2226
info@aacn.org
http://www.aacn.org

American Collegiate Adventures (ACA)

College Courses/Summer Study

American Collegiate Adventures offers high school students the chance to experience and prepare for college during summer vacation. Adventures are based at the University of Wisconsin in Madison; they vary in length from three to six weeks. Participants attend college-level courses taught by university faculty during the week (for college credit or enrichment) and visit regional colleges and recreation sites over the weekend. All students live in comfortable (suite) accommodations, just down the hall from an ACA resident staff member. Courses vary but usually include such basics as "Introduction to Biology" and "Introduction to Chemistry"—perfect for those planning to pursue a degree in health care. Programs in Italy and Spain are also available. Contact ACA for current course listings, prices, and application procedures.

American Collegiate Adventures

1811 West North Avenue, Suite 201
Chicago, IL 60622-0202

800-509-7867
info@acasummer.com
http://www.zfc-consulting.com/
    webprojects/americanadventures

American Holistic Health Association

Membership

The association offers membership ($25) to anyone interested in holistic health. Visit its Web site for more information.

> **American Holistic Health Association**
> PO Box 17400
> Anaheim, CA 92817-7400
> 714-779-6152
> mail@ahha.org
> http://ahha.org

Association of Women's Health, Obstetric and Neonatal Nurses (AWHONN)

Membership

This organization represents nurses who specialize in the care of women and newborns. Its members include neonatal nurses, OB/GYN and labor and delivery nurses, women's health nurses, nurse scientists, nurse executives and managers, childbirth educators, and nurse practitioners. It offers associate membership status for non-nurses who are "involved or interested in women's health, obstetric, or neonatal specialty." Membership benefits include access to AWHONN online forums, subscriptions to *The Journal of Obstetric, Gynecologic and Neonatal Nursing, Every Woman,* and *AWHONN Lifelines,* and the opportunity to partici-pate in the organization's annual conference. Contact the association for more information.

> **Association of Women's Health, Obstetric and Neonatal Nurses**
> 2000 L Street, NW, Suite 740
> Washington, DC 20036-4912
> 800-673-8499
> http://www.awhonn.org

The Center for Excellence in Education

Field Experience

The goal of the Center for Excellence in Education (CEE) is to nurture future leaders in science, technology, and business. And it won't cost you a dime: all of CEE's programs are absolutely free. Since 1984, the CEE has sponsored the Research Science Institute, a six-week residential summer program held at Massachusetts Institute of Technology. Seventy-five high school students with scientific and technological promise are chosen from a field of more than 700 applicants to participate in the program, conducting projects with scientists and researchers. You can read more about specific research projects online.

> **The Center for Excellence in Education**
> 8201 Greensboro Drive, Suite 215
> McLean, VA 22102-3813
> 703-448-9062
> cee@cee.org
> http://www.cee.org

College and Careers Program at the Rochester Institute of Technology

College Course/Summer Study

The Rochester Institute of Technology (RIT) offers its College and Careers Program for rising seniors who want to experience college life and explore career options in science, computing, liberal arts, and other subject areas. The program, founded in 1990, allows you to spend a Friday and Saturday on campus, living in the dorms and attending four sessions on the career areas of your choice. Past science-related sections included Computers in a Science or Pre-Med Track, Medical Ultrasound: Seeing Through Sound, Medical Sciences: Medical Detective—You Make the Call!, Premedical Studies and Biomedical Sciences: What's Up Doc?, Biotechnology/Genetic Engineering: How to Clone a Dinosaur, Bioinformatics: Enabling Discovery, Premedical Studies: So, You Want to Be a Doctor?, and Chemistry: The Wonders of Chemistry. In each session, participants work with RIT students and faculty to gain hands-on experience in the subject area. This residential program is held twice each summer, usually once in mid-July and again in early August. The registration deadline is one week before the start of the program, but space is limited and students are accepted on a first-come, first-served basis. Check the RIT Web site for details about registration. For further information about the program and specific sessions on offer, contact the RIT admissions office.

College and Careers Program
Rochester Institute of Technology
Office of Admissions
60 Lomb Memorial Drive
Rochester, NY 14623-5604
585-475-6631
https://ambassador.rit.edu/
    careers2006/

Early Experience Program at the University of Denver

College Course/Summer Study

The University of Denver invites academically gifted high school students interested in science and other subjects to apply for its Early Experience Program, which involves participating in university-level classes during the school year and especially during the summer. This is a commuter-only program. Interested students must submit a completed application (with essay), official high school transcript, standardized test results (PACT/ACT/PSAT/SAT), a letter of recommendation from a counselor or teacher, and have a minimum GPA of 3.0. Contact the Early Experience Program coordinator for more information, including application forms, available classes, and current fees.

University of Denver
Office of Academic Youth Programs
    Early Experience Program
Attn: Pam Campbell, Coordinator
1981 South University Boulevard
Denver, CO 80210-4209
303-871-2663
pcampbe1@du.edu
http://www.du.edu/education/ces/
    ee.html

Exploration Summer Programs (ESP) at Yale University

College Course/Summer Study

Exploration Summer Programs has been offering academic summer enrichment programs to students for nearly 30 years. Rising high school sophomores, juniors, and seniors can participate in ESP's Senior Program at Yale University. Two three-week residential and day sessions are available and are typically held in June and July. Participants can choose from more than 80 courses in science (such as anatomy and physiology, biomedical ethics, chemistry, and microbiology) and other areas of study. Students entering the 11th or 12th grades can take college seminars, which provide course work that is similar to that of first-year college study. All courses and seminars are ungraded and not-for-credit. In addition to academics, students participate in extracurricular activities such as tours, sports, concerts, weekend recreational trips, college trips, and discussions of current events and other issues. Tuition for the Residential Senior Program is approximately $4,345 for one session and $8,000 for two sessions. Day session tuition ranges from approximately $2,150 for one session to $3,995 for two sessions. A limited number of need-based partial and full scholarships are available. Programs are also available for students in grades four through nine. Contact ESP for more information.

Exploration Summer Programs

470 Washington Street, PO Box 368
Norwood, MA 02062-0368
781-762-7400
http://www.explo.org/senior

Frontiers at Worcester Polytechnic Institute

College Courses/Summer Study

Frontiers is an on-campus research and learning experience for high school students who are interested in science, mathematics, and engineering. Areas of study include biology and biotechnology, mathematics, aerospace engineering, computer science, electrical and computer engineering, mechanical engineering, physics, and robotics. Participants attend classes and do lab work Monday through Friday for two weeks in July. Participants also have the opportunity to try out one of five communication modules: creative writing, elements of writing, music, speech, and theater. In addition to the academic program, participants attend evening workshops, live performances, field trips, movies, and tournaments. Applications are typically available in January and due in March. Tuition is about $2,000; this covers tuition, room, board, linens, transportation, and entrance fees to group activities. A $500 nonrefundable deposit is required. For more information, contact the program director.

Worcester Polytechnic Institute

Frontiers Program
100 Institute Road
Worcester, MA 01609-2280
508-831-5286
frontiers@wpi.edu
http://www.admissions.wpi.edu/
   Frontiers

Health Occupations Students of America (HOSA)

Competition, Conference, Membership

HOSA has been working since 1976 "to promote career opportunities in the health care industry and to enhance the delivery of quality health care to all people." It is an integral part of the health occupations curriculum in its member schools. The organization offers a variety of competitions at the state and national levels. Qualifying HOSA participants compete in a variety of skill, leadership, and related events, including CPR/First Aid, Medical Spelling, Biomedical Debate, Emergency Medical Technician, Medical Math, Medical Terminology, Medical Laboratory Assisting, Physical Therapy, Sports Medicine, First Aid/Rescue Breathing, Personal Care, Practical Nursing, Nursing Assisting, Speaking Skills, Job Seeking Skills, and Interviewing Skills. HOSA also sponsors an annual national conference and also teams with a variety of organizations to offer scholarships. To participate in HOSA events, you must work with your school, so speak to a counselor or teacher about your interest in the organization.

Health Occupations Students of America

6021 Morriss Road, Suite 111
Flower Mound, TX 75028-3764
800-321-HOSA
http://www.hosa.org

High School Honors Program/ Summer Challenge Program at Boston University

College Course/Summer Study

Two summer educational opportunities are available for high school students interested in science and other majors. Rising high school seniors can participate in the High School Honors Program, which offers six-week, for-credit undergraduate study at the university. Students take two for-credit classes (up to eight credits) alongside regular Boston College students, live in dorms on campus, and participate in extracurricular activities and tours of local attractions. Classes can be taken in such subject areas as biochemistry, biology, biomedical-clinical, chemistry, mathematics, physical science, and psychology. The program typically begins in early July. Students who demonstrate financial need may be eligible for financial aid. Tuition for the program is approximately $3,744, with registration/program fees ($350) and room and board options ($1,701 to $1,832) extra. Rising high school sophomores, juniors, and seniors in the University's Summer Challenge Program learn about college life and take college classes in a non-credit setting. The program last two weeks and is offered in three sessions. Students get to choose two seminars (which feature lectures, group and individual work, project-based assignments, and field trips) from a total of eight available programs. Seminar choices include Science, Psychology, Visual Arts, Business, Law, International Politics, Creative Writing, Persuasive Writing, and Boston Studies. Students live in dorms on campus and participate in extracurricular activities and tours of local attractions. The cost of the program is approximately $2,750 (which includes tuition, a room charge, meals, and sponsored activities). Visit the university's Summer Programs Web site for more information.

Boston University Summer Programs

755 Commonwealth Avenue
Boston, MA 02215-1401
617-353-5124
summer@bu.edu
http://www.bu.edu/summer/high_school/index.html

High School Journalism Institute at Indiana University

College Courses/Summer Study

Rising high school sophomores, juniors, and seniors who are interested in careers in writing (including writing about science and medical issues) may participate in the High School Journalism Institute at Indiana University, a five-day residential or commuter program. Workshops are offered in Television News, Yearbook, Newspaper/News Magazine, Business/Advertising, and Photojournalism. Residential participants stay on separate floors (by gender) of Teter Residence Hall, which is air conditioned and within walking distance of most workshop sessions. Cost for the five-day session for resident participants is $295; this includes tuition, residence hall room, and most supplies. Meal debit cards of either $40 or $70 are extra. Commuters pay $250 for the five-day session. Applications are typically due in June. Contact the institute for more information.

Indiana University

High School Journalism Institute
School of Journalism
Bloomington, IN 47405
812-855-0895
ljjohnso@indiana.edu
http://www.journalism.indiana.edu/hsji/students.html

Intel Science Talent Search

Competition

Since 1942, Science Service has held a nationwide competition for talented high school seniors who plan to pursue careers in medicine, science, engineering, and math. Those who win find themselves in illustrious company: former winners have gone on to win Nobel Prizes, National Medals of Science, and MacArthur Foundation fellowships. High school students in the United States and its territories, as well as American students abroad, are eligible to compete for more than $1 million in scholarships and prizes awarded to participants, including the top one for $100,000. If you'd like to enter next year's competition, contact the Talent Search for more information.

Intel Science Talent Search

1719 N Street, NW
Washington, DC 20036-2801
202-785-2255
http://www.sciserv.org/sts

Intern Exchange International, Ltd.

Employment and Internship Opportunities

High school students ages 16 to 18 (including graduating seniors) who are interested in gaining real-life experience in medicine can participate in a month-long summer internship in London, England. Participants will work as interns with hospital and clinic staff at St. Thomas' Hospital, St. Bartholomew's Hospital, or Hammersmith Hospital. There is also a veterinary medicine program. The cost of the program is approximately $6,245, plus airfare; this fee includes tuition, housing (students live in residence halls at the University of London), breakfast and dinner daily, housekeeping service, linens and towels, special dinner events, weekend trips and excursions, group activities including scheduled theater, and a Tube Pass. Contact Intern Exchange International for more information.

Intern Exchange International, Ltd.

2606 Bridgewood Circle
Boca Raton, FL 33434-4118
561-477-2434
info@internexchange.com
http://www.internexchange.com

Junior Scholars Program at Miami University-Oxford

College Courses/Summer Study

Academically talented high school seniors can earn six to eight semester hours of college credit and learn about university life by participating in the Junior Scholars Program at Miami University-Oxford. Students may choose from more than 40 courses, including recent courses such as Microorganisms and Human Disease, Introduction to Psychology, Principles of Human Physiology, and Aging in American Society. In addition to academics, scholars participate in social events, recreational activities, and cocurricular semi-

nars. Program participants live in an air-conditioned residence hall. Fees range from approximately $2,063 to $3,241 depending on the number of credit hours taken and applicant's place of residence (Ohio residents receive a program discount). There is an additional fee of approximately $200 for books. The application deadline is typically in mid-May. Visit the program's Web site for additional eligibility requirements and further details.

Miami University-Oxford

Junior Scholars Program 202
Bachelor Hall
Oxford, OH 45056-3414
513-529-5825
juniorscholars@muohio.edu
http://www.units.muohio.edu/
   jrscholars

Junior Science and Humanities Symposium (JSHS)

Conference

The Junior Science and Humanities Symposium encourages high school students (grades 9 through 12) who are gifted in the sciences, engineering, and mathematics to develop their analytical and creative skills. There are nearly 50 symposia held at locations all around the United States—including Georgetown University, the University of Toledo, and Seattle Pacific University—so that each year some 10,000 students are able to participate. Funded by the U.S. Army Research Office since its inception in 1958 (and by the U.S. Army, Navy, and Air Force since 1995), the JSHS has little to do with the military and everything to do with research. At each individual symposium, researchers and educators from various universities and laboratories meet with the high school students (and some of their teachers) to study new scientific findings, pursue their own interests in the lab, and discuss and debate relevant issues. Participants learn how scientific research can be used to benefit humanity, and they are strongly encouraged to pursue such research in college and as a career. To provide further encouragement, one attendee at each symposium will win a scholarship and the chance to present his or her own research at the national Junior Science and Humanities Symposium. Finalists from each regional JSHS win all-expenses-paid trips to the national symposium, where the top research students can win additional scholarships worth up to $16,000 and trips to the prestigious London International Youth Sciences Forum. For information about the symposium in your region and on eligibility requirements, contact the national Junior Science and Humanities Symposium.

Junior Science and Humanities Symposium (JSHS)
Academy of Applied Science
24 Warren Street
Concord, NH 03301-4048
603-228-4520
phampton@aas-world.org
http://www.jshs.org

Learning for Life Exploring Program
Field Experience
Learning for Life's Exploring Program is a career exploration program that allows

young people to work closely with community organizations to learn life skills and explore careers. Opportunities are available in health and other fields. Each Program has five areas of emphasis: career opportunities, service learning, leadership experience, life skills, and character education. As a participant in the health program, you will work closely with health care professionals and learn about the demands and rewards of careers in the field, including options in clinical laboratory science, dental care, dietary science, health services administration, pharmacy, podiatry, public health, health information and communication, and mental, physical, and social health specialties.

To be eligible to participate in this program, you must have completed the eighth grade and be 14 years old *or* be between the ages of 15 years of age and 20. This program is open to both males and females.

To find a Learning for Life office in your area (there are more than 300 located throughout the United States), contact the Learning for Life Exploring Program.

Learning for Life Exploring Program
1325 West Walnut Hill Lane,
  PO Box 152079
Irving, TX 75015-2079
972-580-2433
http://www.learningforlife.org/
  exploring/health/index.html

Medcamp
Camps
Arizona high school students in their junior and senior years have the oppor-

tunity to attend Medcamp during their summer vacation. The University of Arizona Health Sciences Center (AHSC) has sponsored this free, three-day career camp every July since 1992. High schools around the state nominate one boy and one girl for the program; the nominees may then submit an application and essay, by which the final participants are selected. If you are chosen to attend MedCamp, you will then explore medical careers while living on the University of Arizona campus under the supervision of medical students. During the day, there are classes, laboratory experiences, hospital tours, and opportunities to speak with and watch health care professionals at work. You leave with a better overall understanding of the health care industry and information on specific careers such as nursing, physical and occupational therapy, and pharmacy. If you are interested in attending MedCamp, discuss it with your science teacher, who should receive nomination forms from the AHSC.

Medcamp
University of Arizona Health
　Sciences Center
Office of Public Affairs
1501 North Campbell Avenue,
　PO Box 245095
Tucson, AZ 85724-5095
520-626-7301
riley@u.arizona.edu
http://www.ahsc.arizona.edu/opa/
　medcamp

Medical Application of Science and Health at the Southwest Louisiana Area Health Education Center
Camps
The Southwest Louisiana Area Health Education Center sponsors an annual Medical Application of Science and Health program—known as M*A*S*H—to students entering 10th through 12th grades. This two-week program serves to orient students on different career paths in the health care industry. M*A*S*H students learn how to read throat cultures, conduct EKGs, study college-level biology and medical technology classes, and meet one-on-one with doctors from a range of specialties. After successful completion of the program and exam, students earn three or four hours of college credit, as well as the experience of a lifetime. To be eligible, applicants must have at least a 3.4 GPA. The program is offered at the University of Louisiana-Lafayette and McNeese State University. Visit the organization's Web site for more information on the program.

If this camp sounds interesting, but you don't live in Louisiana, visit the National Area Health Education Center Organization's Web site, http://www.nationala-hec.org/home/index.asp, to see if similar programs are available in your state.

Southwest Louisiana Area Health Education Center
Medical Application of Science and
　Health Program
103 Independence Boulevard
Lafayette, LA 70506-6086
800-435-2432

careers@swlahec.com
http://www.swlahec.com/index.
    php?option=com_content&task=vi
    ew&id=103&Itemid=142

National Area Health Education Center Organization
Camps, Field Experience

The National Area Health Education Center Organization seeks to "enhance access to quality health care, particularly primary and preventive care, by improving the supply and distribution of health care professionals through community/academic educational partnerships." It offers a variety of programs for elementary, middle school, and high school students, including summer health care exploration camps and career presentations. Visit its Web site for an overview of its programs and contact information for affiliates in your state.

**National Area Health Education
Center Organization**
109 VIP Drive, Suite 220
Wexford, PA 15090-6929
888-412-7424
info@nationalahec.org
http://www.nationalahec.org/home/
    index.asp

National Federation of Licensed Practical Nurses (NFLPN)
Membership

The NFLPN is a professional association for licensed practical nurses. Supporters of the federation can apply for membership, which entitles them to subscrip-

tions to organization publications and the opportunity to attend its annual conference, among other benefits. Contact the NFLPN for more information.

**National Federation of Licensed
    Practical Nurses**
605 Poole Drive
Garner, NC 27529-5203
919-779-0046
http://www.nflpn.org

Nursing Camp at Briar Cliff University
Camps

High school juniors and seniors who are considering a career in nursing can learn more about the field by attending Briar Cliff University's summer nursing camp. Attendees participate in clinical experiences, learn first aid and CPR, job-shadow actual nurses, and work closely with Briar Cliff nursing faculty and graduates. Specialty areas of study include emergency room, hospital (medical-surgical), intensive care, labor and delivery, nursery, operating room, pediatrics, and public health. Students who successfully complete the camp earn one hour of college credit. Nursing Camp is held for five days in late June and/or early July. Participants live in a residence hall. Tuition is approximately $265 and covers four nights of lodging, all meals from Monday lunch through Friday lunch, and transportation to clinical experiences and recreational activities. Visit the program's Web site for more information.

Briar Cliff University

Nursing Camp
Attn: Dr. Barbara Condon,
    Chairperson, Department of
    Nursing
3303 Rebecca Street
Sioux City, IA 51104-2324
800-662-3303, ext. 1758
barb.condon@briarcliff.edu
http://www.briarcliff.edu/
    departments/nursing/camp.htm

Nursing Camp at Seattle Pacific University

Camps

High school students who are interested in nursing can attend the Nursing Camp at Seattle Pacific University, a weeklong camp where young people can explore nursing careers and make new friends in the process. Participants can watch nurses in action, become certified in CPR, learn to take blood pressure and pulse, and talk with nursing faculty and recent graduates about the field. Specialty areas include emergency room, home health, intensive care, labor and delivery, nursery, pediatrics, and operating room. Students live in residence halls while attending the camp, which is held in late June. Tuition is approximately $595, and includes lodging, all meals from Sunday dinner through Saturday lunch, and transportation to hospital clinicals and recreation activities. Some financial aid is available. The application deadline is typically in late April. Visit the Web site listed below for more information.

Seattle Pacific University

School of Health Sciences
Nursing Camp
3307 Third Avenue West, Suite 106
Seattle, WA 98119-1922
206-281-2233
http://www.spu.edu/nursing/
    nursingcamp

Pre-College Program at Johns Hopkins University

College Courses/Summer Study

Johns Hopkins University welcomes academically talented high school students to its summertime Pre-College Program. Participants in this program live on Hopkins' Homewood campus for five weeks beginning in early July. They pursue one of 27 programs leading to college credit; those interested in health care should strongly consider enrolling in the Biology or the History of Science and Technology Program. Recent courses included "Introduction to Biological Molecules," which surveys the important structures and functions of macromolecules involved in biological processes, and "Modern Medicine: A Historical Introduction," a scientific and historical look at medicine from the Renaissance to today. Course work is supplemented with presentations by research scientists, laboratory tours, and visits to the famous Johns Hopkins Hospital and Medical School. All participants in the Pre-College Program also attend workshops on college admissions, time management, and diversity. Students who live in the greater Baltimore area have the option of commuting. Contact the Office of Summer Programs for financial aid information, costs, and deadlines. As of July 1, applicants must be at least 15 years old, have completed their sophomore, junior, or senior year, and have a minimum GPA of 3.0 (or "B" average). All applicants must submit an application form, essay, transcript, two recommendations, and a non-refundable application fee (rates vary by date of submission). For more information, including an application form, contact the Office of Summer Programs.

Johns Hopkins University
Office of Summer Programs
Pre-College Program
Wyman Park Building, Suite G4
3400 North Charles Street
Baltimore, MD 21218-2685
800-548-0548
summer@jhu.edu
http://www.jhu.edu/~sumprog/index.html

Science Is Fun! Camp at Miami University of Ohio
Camp
The Center for Chemical Education at Miami University of Ohio sponsors a series of Terrific Science Camps each summer. Area third through seventh graders are welcome to attend the Science Is Fun! Camp. It lasts three hours every day for one week during the month of July. As a participant, you explore the fascinating world of science. The cost for this commuter camp is approximately $100, and free tuition is available to students truly in need of financial aid. Admission is made on a first-come, first-served basis, so you should apply well before the deadline in late April. For an application form and more information on this year's camp, contact Terrific Science Programs.

Miami University Middletown
Terrific Science Programs
Attn: Kitty Blattner
200 Levey Hall
Middletown, OH 45052
513-727-3318
http://www.units.muohio.edu/continuingeducation/summer/youth_programs/youth.htmlx

Science Olympiad
Competition
The Science Olympiad is a national competition based in schools. School teams feed into regional and state tournaments, and the winners at the state level go on to the national competition. Some schools have many teams, all of which compete in their state Science Olympiad. Only one team per school, however, is allowed to represent its state at the national contest, and each state gets a slot. There are four divisions of Science Olympiad: Division A1 and A2 for younger students, Division B for grades six through nine, and Division C for grades nine through twelve. There is no national competition for Division A.

A school team membership fee must be submitted with a completed membership form 30 days before your regional or state tournament. The fee entitles your school to a copy of the Science Olympiad Coaches and Rules Manual plus the eligibility to have up to 15 students at the first level of your state or regional contest. Fees vary from state to state. The

National Science Olympiad is held in a different site every year, and your school team is fully responsible for transportation, lodging, and food.

Specific rules have been developed for each event and must be read carefully. There are numerous different events in each division. You and your teammates can choose the events you want to enter and prepare yourselves accordingly. Winners receive medals, trophies, and some scholarships.

For a list of all Science Olympiad state directors and a membership form, go to the Science Olympiad Web site. You can also write or call the national office for information.

Science Olympiad Inc.
2 Trans Am Plaza Drive, Suite 415
Oakbrook Terrace, IL 60181-4290
630-792-1251
http://www.soinc.org

Secondary Student Training Program (SSTP) at the University of Iowa

College Course/Summer Study

The University of Iowa invites those who have completed grade 10 or 11 to apply to its Secondary Student Training Program (SSTP). The program allows students to explore a particular area of science or health care—such as microbiology, internal medicine, or pathology, pediatrics, or surgery—while experiencing the career field of scientific research. Participants work with university faculty in one of the many laboratories on campus, studying and conducting research projects for approximately 40 hours per week. At the end of the program, which lasts six weeks, you present your project to a formal gathering of faculty, staff, and fellow SSTP participants. Throughout the program you also take part in various seminars on career choices and the scientific profession, and a variety of recreational activities designed especially for SSTP participants. Students live in University of Iowa dormitories and use many of the facilities on campus. The admissions process is highly competitive and is based on an essay, transcript, and recommendations. Those who complete the program have the option of receiving college credit from the University of Iowa. Applications are due by mid-March, and applicants will be notified of the decisions by mid-May. Tuition fees, room, and board generally total around $2,000; spending money and transportation to and from the university are not included. Financial aid is available. For an application form, financial aid information, and to discuss possible research projects, contact the Secondary Student Training Program.

Secondary Student Training Program
E203 Seashore Hall
Iowa City, IA 52242-1316
800-553-4692, ext. 5-3876
william-swain@uiowa.edu
http://www.uiowa.edu/~provost/oi/sstp

SkillsUSA

Competitions

SkillsUSA offers "local, state and national competitions in which students demonstrate occupational and leadership skills." Students who participate in its SkillsUSA Championships can compete in categories such as Basic Health Care Skills, First Aid/CPR, Health Knowledge Bowl, Health Occupations Professional Portfolio, Nurse Assisting, and Practical Nursing. SkillsUSA works directly with high schools and colleges, so ask your guidance counselor or teacher if it is an option for you. Visit the SkillsUSA Web site for more information.

SkillsUSA
PO Box 3000
Leesburg, VA 20177-0300
703-777-8810
http://www.skillsusa.org

Summer College for High School Students at Cornell University
College Course/Summer Study

As part of its Summer College for High School Students, Cornell University offers two medicine and health professions seminars for high school students who have completed their junior or senior years: Body, Mind, and Health: Perspectives for Future Medical Professionals and Biological Research and Health Professions. The Summer College session runs for six weeks from late June until early August. It is largely a residential program designed to acquaint you with all aspects of college life. The Medicine and Health Professions seminars are just two of several such seminars offered by Cornell to allow students to survey various disciplines within the field and interact with working professionals. The seminar meets several times per week and includes lectures and field trips to research laboratories, clinicians' offices, and surgery suites. In addition, Summer College participants take college-level courses of their own choosing. You must bear in mind that these are regular undergraduate courses condensed into a very short time span, so they are especially challenging and demanding. Besides the course material, you will learn time-management and study skills to prepare you for a program of undergraduate study. The university awards letter grades and full undergraduate credit for the courses you complete. Residents live and eat on campus, and enjoy access to the university's recreational facilities and special activities. Academic fees total around $3,400, while housing, food, and recreation fees amount to an additional $1,600. Books, travel, and an application fee are extra. A very limited amount of financial aid is available. Applications are due in early May, although Cornell advises that you submit them well in advance of the deadline; those applying for financial aid must submit their applications by early April. Further information and details of the application procedure are available from the Summer College office.

Cornell University
Summer College for High School
  Students
B20 Day Hall
Ithaca, NY 14853-2801
607-255-6203
http://www.sce.cornell.edu/sc/
  explorations/medicine.php

Summer College for High School Students at Syracuse University

College Course/Summer Study

The Syracuse University Summer College for High School Students features the following programs for those who have just completed their sophomore, junior, or senior year: Engineering and Computer Science, Public Communications, and Liberal Arts/Arts and Sciences. The Summer College lasts six weeks and offers a residential option so participants can experience campus life while still in high school. The program has several aims: to introduce you to the many possible majors and study areas within this general area; to help you match your aptitudes with possible careers; and to prepare you for college, both academically and socially. Students attend classes, listen to lectures, and take field trips to destinations that are related to their specific area of interest. All students are required to take two courses during the program and they receive college credit if they successfully complete the courses. Admission is competitive and is based on recommendations, test scores, and transcripts. The total cost of the residential program is about $5,600; the commuter option costs about $4,375. Some scholarships are available. The application deadline is in mid-May, or mid-April for those seeking financial aid. For further information, contact the Summer College.

Syracuse University
Summer College for High School
    Students
111 Waverly Avenue, Suite 240
Syracuse, NY 13244-2320
315-443-5297
summcoll@syr.edu
http://summercollege.syr.edu

Summer Program for Secondary School Students at Harvard University

College Course/Summer Study

High school students who have completed their sophomore, junior, or senior year may apply to Harvard's Summer Program for Secondary School Students. Students who live on campus take either two four-unit courses or one eight-unit course for college credit. Commuting students may take only one four-unit course for college credit. Recent science-related courses included Introductory Biology, Principles of Genetics, Introduction to Immunology, General Chemistry, and Organic Chemistry. In addition to academics, students can participate in extracurricular activities such as intramural sports, a trivia bowl, a talent show, and dances. Tuition for the program ranges from $2,200 (per four-unit course) to $4,400 (per eight-unit course). A nonrefundable registration fee ($50), health insurance ($110), and room and board ($3,875) are extra. The application deadline for this program is mid-June. Contact the program for more information.

Harvard University
Summer Program for Secondary
    School Students
51 Brattle Street
Cambridge, MA 02138-3701
617-495-3192

ssp@hudce.harvard.edu
http://www.summer.harvard.edu

Summer Science and Engineering Program at Smith College

College Courses/Summer Study

Female high school students who are interested in careers in medicine, science, or engineering can participate in Smith College's Science and Engineering Program. Students in this month-long residential program take either two two-week-long research courses or one four-week-long research course. Recent courses included Women and Exercise: A Biochemical Investigation; Population Biology: An Introduction to the Genetics and Ecology of Natural Populations; and Your Genes, Your Chromosomes: A Laboratory in Human Genetics. Participants give two oral presentations about their work, one at the midpoint of the program and one at the conclusion of the program. In their free time, students participate in a variety of extracurricular activities, such as sports, nature walks, movie nights, museum tours, and cultural activities. For more information on the program, contact the director of Educational Outreach.

Smith College
Summer Science and Engineering
  Program
Attn: Gail E. Scordilis, Ph.D., Director
Educational Outreach
Clark Hall
Northampton, MA 01063-6353
413-585-3060
gscordil@smith.edu
http://www.smith.edu/
  summerprograms/ssep

Summer Study Program at Pennsylvania State University

College Course/Summer Study

High school students who are interested in science and other fields can apply to participate in Penn State's Summer Study programs. The six-and-a-half-week College Credit Program begins in late June and recently offers the following health care-related classes: Introduction to Biobehavioral Health; Human Body: Form and Function; Genetics, Ecology and Evolution; Structure and Functions of Organisms; Introduction to Health Services Organization; Intro to Human Development and Family Studies; Infant and Child Development; Adolescent Development; and Introductory Principles of Nutrition. Students typically choose one college credit course (for three or four credits) and either an enrichment class/workshop or the Kaplan SAT prep class. Students who have completed the 10th, 11th, and 12th grades are eligible to apply. The three-and-a-half-week Non-Credit Enrichment Program is held in July and recently featured science-related classes such as Paging Dr. (Your Name Here): Careers & Trends in Healthcare; Health and Wellness; Journalism/Communications; and Beauty and the Beast: Health and Wellness. Students who have completed the 9th, 10th, and 11th grades are eligible for the program. Tuition for the College Credit Program is approximately $6,195, while tuition for the Non-Credit Enrichment Program is approximately $4,000. Limited financial aid is available. Contact the program for more information.

Pennsylvania State University
Summer Study Program
900 Walt Whitman Road
Melville, NY 11747-2293
800-666-2556
info@summerstudy.com
http://www.summerstudy.com/
    pennstate

Summer Youth Programs at Michigan Technological University
College Course/Summer Study

Michigan Technological University (MTU) offers the Summer Youth Program for students in grades 6 through 11. Participants attend one of four weeklong sessions usually held during the months of July or August, choosing either to commute or to live on campus. Students undertake an "exploration" in one of many career fields—including health care/science—through field trips and discussions with MTU faculty and other professionals. Science classes recently offered included Careers in Health and Fitness; Chemistry; Clinical Laboratory Sciences; Genetic Engineering; Medical Physiology; and Microbiology. The cost of the Summer Youth Program is approximately $525 for the residential option, $325 for commuters. Applications are accepted up to one week before the program begins.

Michigan Technological University
Summer Youth Program
Youth Programs Office, Alumni House
1400 Townsend Drive
Houghton, MI 49931-1295

906-487-2219
http://youthprograms.mtu.edu

Wisconsin Area Health Education Center (AHEC)
Camps

The Wisconsin Area Health Education Center offers four- to six-day summer camps for Wisconsin high school students who are interested in learning more about health care careers. Students participate in hands-on activities conducted by health profession students, instructors, and health care professionals. AHEC and other sponsors cover meals, lodging, and other program costs. A $35 reservation fee is required. Scholarships are available for those with financial need. For more information, visit the Wisconsin AHEC's Web site.

If this camp sounds interesting, but you don't live in Wisconsin, visit the National Area Health Education Center Organization's Web site, http://www.nationala-hec.org/home/index.asp, to see if similar programs are available in your state.

Wisconsin Area Health Education Center
1300 University Avenue, 203 Bradley Memorial
Madison, WI 53706-1510
608-263-1712
http://www.ahec.wisc.edu/
    SumCamps.html

Women in the Sciences and Engineering (WISE) Week at Pennsylvania State University
Camp

The Pennsylvania State University (Penn State) offers a Women in the Sciences and Engineering (WISE) Week program in June for female rising juniors and seniors. Participants are academically talented, with strong math and science skills, headed for college, and considering career paths in health, science, and engineering. Students apply to one WISE option, either Sciences or Engineering. Competition is considerable as only 36 young women are accepted into each option. Accommodation is in a campus residence hall with collegiate women as your supervisors. The cost of the program is about $375, which covers everything except transportation to and from Penn State's University Park Campus; a limited number of need-based scholarships are available. A completed application form, one letter of recommendation, an essay, any recent standardized test scores, and a current high school transcript must be submitted by the beginning of April. Members of minority groups and students with physical disabilities are strongly encouraged to apply. For further information about WISE Week and the application process, contact the program.

Pennsylvania State University
Women in the Sciences and
    Engineering Week
319 Boucke Building
University Park, PA 16802
814-865-3342
wise@psu.edu
http://www.equity.psu.edu/wise/
    wisecamp.asp

Young Scholars Program at the University of Maryland
College Course/Summer Study

The Young Scholars Program is sponsored by the University of Maryland for motivated juniors and seniors. Participants in the three-week program explore the fields of biology, business/entrepreneurship, journalism, kinesiology, public health, and other areas and take a college-level course. College credit is awarded to students who satisfactorily complete the course. Participants commute or live in the residence halls at the University of Maryland and take their meals on campus or in selected College Park restaurants. To apply, you must submit an application form, an essay, two letters of recommendations, a current transcript, and an application fee of $55 by mid-May. Admissions decisions are based primarily on the recommendations, a GPA of 3.0 or better, and overall academic ability. Cost for this program is $2,719 for the residential option and $1,719 for the commuter option. For further details and an application form, visit the Web site below or contact the Summer Sessions and Special Programs staff.

University of Maryland
Summer Sessions and Special
    Programs
Mitchell Building, 1st Floor
College Park, MD 20742
301-314-8240
http://www.summer.umd.edu/
    youngscholars

Read a Book

When it comes to finding out about health care, don't overlook books. (You're reading one now, after all.) What follows is a short, annotated list of books and periodicals related to health care. The books range from personal accounts of what it's like to be a health care professional, to career and test preparation guides. Don't be afraid to check out the professional health care journals, either. The technical stuff may be way above your head right now, but if you take the time to become familiar with one or two, you're bound to pick up some of what is important to doctors, nurses, and other health care professionals, not to mention begin to feel like a part of their world, which is what you're interested in, right?

We've tried to include recent materials as well as old favorites. Always check for the most recent editions, and, if you find an author you like, ask your librarian to help you find more. Keep reading good books!

❏ BOOKS

Alley, Michael. *The Craft of Scientific Writing.* New York: Springer, 1997. A reference tool for science writers at all levels of professional experience, this textbook provides practical examples of the dos and don'ts of science writing. Students will learn how to write about science in a concise, engaging manner so that they reach their audience—whether it is other scientists or the general public.

Baker, Diane L., et al. (eds.). *A Guide to Genetic Counseling.* New York: Wiley-Liss Inc., 1998. Written for individuals interested in or studying to become genetic counselors, this book explores the multidimensional facets of this emerging field. Case studies and real-world practitioners provide the substance for this first book of its kind.

Barnum, Barbara Stevens. *Spirituality in Nursing: From Traditional to New Age.* New York: Springer Publishing Company, 2003. Gives a thorough and accessible overview of spirituality, cast as a component of nursing theory and practice. Addresses such major nursing issues as healing, religion, ethics, disease, and death.

Burkhardt, Margaret A., and Alvita K. Nathaniel. *Ethics And Issues In Contemporary Nursing.* 2d ed. Stamford, Conn.: Thomson Delmar Learning, 2001. This book covers ethical issues in the nursing professions, and gives models on how to make these important decisions.

Canfield, Jack, Mark Victor Hansen, Mary Mitchell-Autio, and LeAnn

Thieman. *Chicken Soup for the Nurse's Soul: 101 Stories to Celebrate, Honor and Inspire the Nursing Profession.* Deerfield Beach, Fla.: HCI, 2001. An inspiring and entertaining collection of short stories celebrating nurses and their heroic work.

Cardillo, Donna. *Your First Year as a Nurse: Making the Transition from Total Novice to Successful Professional.* Three Rivers, Minn.: Three Rivers Press, 2001. Survival tips on how to succeed as a nurse. Much of this author's research is based on actual interviews with both new and seasoned nurses in the United States and Canada.

Carr, Joseph J., and John M. Brown. *Introduction to Biomedical Equipment Technology.* 4th ed. Upper Saddle River, N.J.: Prentice Hall, 2000. This textbook offers an in-depth look at the technology involved in developing today's most complex electronic medical equipment.

Catalano, Joseph T. *Nursing Now: Today's Issues, Tomorrow's Trends.* 3d ed. Philadelphia, Penn.: F.A. Davis Company, 2002. Discusses models of nursing, ethical dilemmas, cultural diversity, leadership, as well as other issues important to the field of nursing.

Croft, Jennifer. *Careers in Midwifery.* New York: Rosen Publishing Group, 1995. An overview of the history of midwifery, the categories of certification and training, birth settings, and career planning. Addresses midwives versus traditional heath care debate.

Eliopoulos, Charlotte. *Gerontological Nursing.* 5th ed. Philadelphia, Penn.: Lippincott Williams & Wilkins, 2000. An accessible and comprehensive basic gerontology text, focusing on health promotion and self-care. Clear, concise, and practically oriented, this text is the perfect guide to understanding and meeting the challenges of providing services to elderly patients in a variety of settings.

Ferri, Fred F. *Practical Guide to the Care of the Medical Patient.* 5th ed. Philadelphia, Penn.: W.B. Saunders Company, 2001. This pocket manual for medical students contains easy-to-find medical diagnoses and treatment options for a wide spectrum of medical conditions. It serves as a useful reference tool for students doing clinical rotations or studying for internal medicine exams.

Frederickson, Keville. *Opportunities in Nursing Careers.* 2d ed. New York: McGraw-Hill Companies, 2003. Offers good vocational guidance for a variety of nursing careers, exploring the financial benefits of each.

Friedman, Marilyn M. *Family Nursing: Research, Theory, and Practice.* 4th ed. Upper Saddle River, N.J.: Prentice Hall, 2002. A thorough survey of the educational requirements, procedures, and vicissitudes of family nursing.

Goldsmith, Seth B. *Principles of Health Care Management: Compliance Consumerism and Accountability in the 21st Century.* Sudbury, Mass.: Jones & Bartlett Publishers, 2005. Students interested in learning about the U.S. health care system and the managerial aspects of working within such a system will find this a thorough book, full of relevant case studies.

Harper, Peter S. *Practical Genetic Counseling.* New York: Hodder Arnold Publication, 1998. As scientific discoveries about human genetic disorders continue to be uncovered, this book details the work that must be done by genetic counselors and others in the medical field to make meaningful use of new information. The book contains a listing of the most common genetic disorders, useful to anyone researching a disorder or studying to work in the field of genetics.

Hegner, Barbara, Barbara Acello, and Esther Caldwell. *Nursing Assistant: A Nursing Process Approach.* 9th ed. Stamford, Conn.: Thomson Delmar Learning, 2003. Covers important knowledge and skills needed by nursing assistants. Also includes a step-by-step guide to more than 160 common procedures.

Iles, Robert L. *Guidebook to Better Medical Writing.* Revised ed. Olathe, Kans.: Iles Publications, 2003. This straightforward guidebook provides basic advice to students and medical professionals about developing an appropriate writing style within the genre of medical writing.

Iyer, Patricia W. *Legal Nurse Consulting: Principles and Practices.* 2d ed. Boca Raton, Fla.: CRC Press, 2002. An important reference to the growing field of legal nurse consulting. Gives practical information for the many practice opportunities for legal nurse consultants.

Kasper, Dennis L., et al. *Harrison's Principles of Internal Medicine.* 16th ed. New York: McGraw-Hill, 2004. This all-encompassing medical textbook covers every aspect of internal medicine—from diseases to diagnosis to treatment. Viewed as the authoritative, must-have book by many medical professionals and students, this newly updated book provides up-to-date, highly valuable medical information.

Katz, Janet R., Carol J. Carter, Joyce Bishop, and Sarah Lyman Kravits. *Keys to Nursing Success.* 2d ed. Upper Saddle River, N.J.: Prentice Hall, 2003. Gives students insight and advice for a career as a nurse.

Leonard, Peggy C. *Building a Medical Vocabulary.* 5th ed. St. Louis, Miss.: Mosby, 2003. Excellent guide to the language of health care. Teaches the fundamental word parts that are used as the "building blocks" of more complicated terminology.

Lippincott Williams & Wilkins. *Critical Care Nursing Made Incredibly Easy!* Philadelphia, Penn.: Lippincott Williams & Wilkins, 2003. Illustrated, detailed book on almost 100 critical care disorders. This book also reviews steps involved in common nursing procedures, such as interpreting results, dispensing medicine, and nursing intervention.

———. *Illustrated Handbook of Nursing Care.* Philadelphia, Penn.: Lippincott Williams & Wilkins, 1998. Addresses every key nursing topic, and contains more than 500 illustrations along with charts and sample documentation forms. A comprehensive guide to the ins and outs of the nursing process.

———. *Nursing 2006 Drug Handbook.* 26th ed. Philadelphia, Penn.: Lippincott Williams & Wilkins, 2005. Includes information on newly approved drugs, their effectiveness, interactions with other medicines, and length of effectiveness. Also features a chapter that covers Spanish-English drug translations, cross references, and a companion mini CD.

———. *Pediatric Nursing Made Incredibly Easy!* Philadelphia, Penn.: Lippincott Williams & Wilkins, 2000. Covers growth and development of children. Includes step-by-step procedure instructions, quizzes, and study guides.

McCarthy, Claire. *Everyone's Child: A Pediatrician's Story of an Inner-City Practice.* New York: Scribner, 2002. This chronicle of one doctor's experiences working in an inner-city clinic serves as a guidebook for anyone interested in serving as a medical practitioner to the underprivileged in the United States. The author, of upper-middle class background herself, shares what she has learned not only about practicing medicine in such a setting, but about the people she treats.

McKinney, Anne. *Real-Resumes for Nursing Jobs: Including Real Resumes Used to Change Careers and Resumes Used to Gain Federal Employment.* Fayetteville, N.C.: Prep Publishing, 2003. This book gives tips on how to create a winning resume—perfect for new grads or those interested in crossing over to other health care fields. Also includes examples of actual resumes and helpful information on obtaining federal government jobs.

Novotny, Jeanne M., Doris T. Lippman, Nicole K. Sanders, and Joyce J. Fitzpatrick. *101 Careers in Nursing.* New York: Springer Publishing Company, 2003. This book gives a quick overview of 101 different nursing careers, as well as their education requirements and compensation ranges. Also includes a chapter on career searches and certification.

Pagliarulo, Michael A. *Introduction to Physical Therapy.* 2d ed. St. Louis, Miss.: C.V. Mosby, 2001. This beginners-level textbook introduces students to terminology in the field as well as the job functions of those employed in physical therapy. The book also details the therapies that practitioners use to treat patients with disorders in various bodily systems.

Peterson, Veronica. *Just the Facts: A Pocket Guide to Nursing.* St. Louis, Miss.: Mosby, 2002. A quick and easy reference for beginning nursing students, filled with charts, graphs, outlines, and easy-to-read tables.

Potter, Patricia A., and Anne Griffin Perry. *Fundamentals of Nursing.* 6th ed. St. Louis, Miss.: Mosby, 2004. An important resource for nursing students that includes care plans and a CD-ROM supplement.

Sherry, Clifford. *Opportunities in Medical Imaging Careers.* New York: McGraw-Hill, 2000. This resource book defines the opportunities that exist in medical imaging careers for students who are considering the field. Readers will find the book full of definitions, facts, figures, and statistical information.

Slatt, Lisa M., et al. *Essentials of Family Medicine.* 4th ed. Philadelphia, Penn.: Lippincott Williams & Wilkins, 2002. This reference book for medical students serves as an introduction to what it means to practice family medicine. Sections on the principles of family medicine, preventative care, and common problems are each covered with an evidence-based approach.

Smith, Sandra F., Donna Duell, and Barbara Martin. *Clinical Nursing Skills: Basic to Advanced.* 6th ed. Upper Saddle River, N.J.: Prentice Hall, 2003. This textbook is written for all levels of nursing, from new to advanced. Offers 650 new and updated skills as well as a chapter on bioterrorism.

Sorrentino, Sheila A., and Bernie Gorek. *Mosby's Essentials for Nursing Assistants.* 2d ed. St. Louis, Miss.: Mosby, 2001. Covers the fundamental skills needed to be a nursing assistant. This edition includes more than 500 color illustrations.

Sparks, Sheila M., and Cynthia M. Taylor. *Nursing Diagnosis Reference Manual.* 5th ed. Philadelphia, Penn.: Lippincott Williams & Wilkins, 2001. Important guide for creating care plans—from pediatric to geriatric.

Springhouse Publishing. *Maternal-Neonatal Nursing Made Incredibly Easy!* Los Angeles, Cal.: Springhouse Publishing, 2003. Covers all aspects of maternal-neonatal nursing. CD-ROM supplement includes quizzes, exam review, and NCLEX preparation tips.

———. *Medical-Surgical Nursing Made Incredibly Easy!* Los Angeles, Cal.: Springhouse Publishing, 2003. A great book for medical-surgical nursing students, including those reviewing for NCLEX exams. Includes discussion of more than 300 disorders, with quizzes, illustrations, tables, and other study guides.

———. *Psychiatric Nursing Made Incredibly Easy!* Los Angeles, Cal.: Springhouse Publishing, 2003. Covers more than 70 psychiatric conditions, including their diagnosis and different treatment options.

Swick, Sandra, and Corrine Grimes. *Barron's How to Prepare for the Nursing School Entrance Exams.* 2d ed. Hauppauge, N.Y.: Barron's Educational Series, 2004. Provides a great review for the exam. Gives subject reviews and a full-length model test.

Thibeault, Stephanie. *Stressed Out About Nursing School! An Insider's Guide to Success.* Orlando, Fla.: Bandido Books, 2001. What to expect before, during, and after, nursing school—all from a student's point of view.

Tierney, Lawrence M., et al (eds.). *Current Medical Diagnosis and Treatment 2006.* New York: McGraw-Hill Medical, 2005. This well-respected—and lengthy—publication offers diagnosis and treatment information on more than 1,000 of the most common diseases, in every major division of medicine. Those who purchase the book will also receive access to an online version.

Vallano, Annette. *Your Career In Nursing: Manage Your Future in the Changing World of Healthcare.* New York: Kaplan, 2003. This book is important reading for those interested in career mobility within the nursing field. Special chapters address the career environment for male nurses, as well as second-career nurses.

Weishapple, Cynthia. *Introduction to Legal Nurse Consulting.* Stamford, Conn.: Thomson Delmar Learning, 2000. Important resource for nurses considering a career in legal consulting. Includes career profiles and advice from successful legal nurse consultants.

Young, Audrey. *What Patients Taught Me: A Medical Student's Journey.* Seattle, Wash.: Sasquatch Books, 2004. This autobiographical book chronicles the experiences of a young medical student as she moves from working with rural populations in the United States, to South Africa, and back to the U.S., working with refugees and the homeless. Focusing on the human element of medicine, it portrays medicine as an intensely rewarding, yet extremely difficult, field.

❏ PERIODICALS

Advance for LPNs. Published biweekly in print and online versions by Merion Publications (2900 Horizon Drive, King of Prussia, PA 19406-2651, 800-355-5627). Provides information on issues of interest to licensed practical nurses, book reviews, job listings, and career advice. Visit http://lpn.advance-web.com to read sample articles.

Advance for Nurse Practitioners. Published monthly by Merion Publications (2900 Horizon Drive, King of Prussia, PA 19406-2651, 800-355-5627). Provides information on clinical issues, industry developments, jobs, and salaries. Read sample articles at http://www.advancefornp.com.

American College of Obstetricians and Gynecologists Clinical Review. This bimonthly online newsletter, available to American College of Obstetricians and Gynecologists (409 12th Street, SW, PO Box 96920, Washington, DC 20090-6920, 202-638-5577, resources@acog.org, http://www.acog.org/navbar/current/publications.cfm) members, summarizes developments in the field and emerging issues. The yearly review of the annual board certification exam provides essential information to graduating medical students.

American Family Physician. Published biweekly by the American Academy of Family Physicians (11400 Tomahawk Creek Parkway, Leawood, KS 66211-2672, 800-274-2237, afpcirc@aafp.org, http://www.aafp.org/afp.xml), this scholarly journal for medical professionals contains articles on recent research findings, the latest news in the field, editorials, and more. Visit the its Web site to read sample articles.

American Journal of Critical Care. Published bimonthly by the American Association of Critical-Care Nurses (PO Box 611, Holmes, PA 19043-9873, 800-345-8112, ajcc@aacn.org, http://ajcc.aacnjournals.org). Offers clinical studies, research studies, case reports, reports on new apparatus and techniques, reviews, and guest editorials.

American Journal of Human Genetics. This monthly professional journal of the American Society of Human Genetics American (Brigham and Women's Hospital, New Research Building, Room 160A, 77 Avenue Louis Pasteur, Boston, MA 02115-5727, 617-525-4770, ajhg@ajhg.net, http://www.journals.uchicago.edu/AJHG) serves professionals in a broad range of medical fields that are affected by genetics-related research. It provides the latest news and discoveries in the realm of hereditary disorders.

American Journal of Nursing. Published monthly by Lippincott Williams & Wilkins (PO Box 1620, Hagerstown, MD 21741-1620, 800-638-3030, http://www.lww.com). An important and influential magazine, containing compelling articles and editorials, photo essays, and medical essays.

American Medical Writers Association Journal. Published quarterly by the American Medical Writers Association (40 West Gude Drive, Suite 101, Rockville, MD 20850-1192, 301-294-5303, amwa@amwa.org, http://www.amwa.org/default/publications/journal.asp), this resource for medical writers provides timely information on goings-on in the field along with information on the latest opportunities for experienced medical writers.

The American Nurse. Published bimonthly by the American Nurses Association (8515 Georgia Avenue, Suite 400, Silver Spring, MD 20910-3492, 800-637-0323, http://www.nursingworld.org/tan). Covers a wide variety of topics that are important to nurses in the United States, including nursing shortages and practice issues. A student discount is available to subscribers.

Annals of Family Medicine. This bimonthly research journal (Circulation Department, 11400 Tomahawk Creek Parkway, Leawood, KS 66211-2672, 800-274-2237, ext. 5164, AnnFamMed@case.edu, http://www.annfammed.org) provides thought-provoking articles on the latest research and issues in family medicine. The topics covered are not only critical to medical professionals' ability to stay on top of the latest medical developments, but also highly interesting to anyone interested in medical research. Sample articles are available online.

Biomedical Instrumentation and Technology. Published bimonthly by the Association for the Advancement of Medical Instrumentation (1110 North Glebe Road, Suite 220, Arlington, VA 22201-4795, 800-332-2264, ext. 217, webmaster@aami.org, http://www.aami.org/publications/BIT/index.html), this peer-reviewed journal for anyone involved with medical instrumentation and technology contains articles pertaining to trends in the field, safety and regulatory issues, and practical information on administrative and equipment-related topics.

Critical Care Nurse. Published bimonthly by the American Association of Critical-Care Nurses (PO Box 611, Holmes, PA 19043-9873, 800-345-8112, ccn@aacn.org, http://ccn.aacnjournals.org). Seeks to provide critical care nurses with information about the bedside care of critically and acutely ill patients, as well as practice issues.

Dermatology Insights. Published biannually by the American Academy of Dermatology (930 East Woodfield Road, Schaumburg, IL 60173-4729, 847-330-0230, MRC@aad.org, http://www.aad.org/public/Publications/derminsights.htm), this magazine provides articles of interest not only to dermatologists, but also to anyone afflicted with a skin, hair, or nail condition. Sample issues can be accessed online, and recent articles cover such varied topics as diaper rash, psoriasis, melanoma, and tattooing.

Genetics Online. This monthly research journal published by the Genetics Society of America (9650 Rockville Pike, Bethesda, MD 20814-3998, 301-634-7300, http://www.genetics.org) contains scholarly articles of interest to medical professionals working in a field of genetics. The articles are complex and technical in nature, and probably not accessible to the layperson.

Healthcare Executive. Published bimonthly by the Foundation of the American College of Healthcare Executives (Department 77-72069, Chicago, IL 60678-2069, 312-424-9456, http://www.ache.org/pubs/hcexecsub.cfm), this magazine covers issues of importance to those working on the business end of the health care industry. The publication includes articles written by experts in the field as well as interviews with hospital administrators. Articles cover such topics as facility management, technology trends, and diversity in the workplace.

Home Healthcare Nurse. Published monthly by Lippincott Williams & Wilkins (PO Box 1620, Hagerstown, MD 21741-1620, 800-638-3030, http://www.homehealthcarenurseonline.com). Probably the most thorough journal of home health care nursing, providing strategies for assessing the health of homebound patients, and also for dealing with terminal illness, depression, and death.

Journal of Allergy and Clinical Immunology. Published monthly by the American Academy of Allergy, Asthma & Immunology (555 East Wells Street, Suite 1100 Milwaukee, WI 53202-3823, 414-272-6071, info@aaaai.org, http://www.aaaai.org/members/jaci.stm), this scientific journal, accessible online to subscribers only, includes the latest research studies completed by doctors and scientists specializing in allergy and immunology.

Journal of Diagnostic Medical Sonography. Published bimonthly by the Society of Diagnostic Medical Sonography (PO Box 200971, Dallas, TX 75320-0971, 214-473-8057, http://www.sdms.org/jdms/default.asp), this research journal, accessible online to members only, contains research studies along with case studies, book reviews, and more. Members can also attain continuing education credit by reading a designated article each month and completing an online test.

Journal of Legal Nurse Consulting. Published quarterly by the American Association of Legal Nurse Consultants (401 North Michigan Avenue, Chicago, IL 60611-4255, jlnc@aalnc.org, http://www.aalnc.org/edu-pro/journal.cfm). Offers a variety of articles about medical-legal issues, including managed care, medical and products liability issues, life care planning, and forensics, as well as business advice and networking hints.

Journal of Neuroscience Nursing. Published bimonthly by the American Association of Neuroscience Nurses (4700 West Lake Avenue, Glenview, IL 60025-1485, http://www.aann.org/journal). One of only two journals in the world specializing in neuroscience nursing; written and reviewed by practicing nurses.

Journal of Nursing Education. Published monthly by Slack Incorporated (6900 Grove Road, Thorofare, NJ 08086-9447, 856-848-1000, customerservice@slackinc.com, http://www.journalofnursingeducation.com).

Offers original articles and ideas for nursing educators.

Journal of Obstetric, Gynecologic and Neonatal Nursing. Published bimonthly (on behalf of the Association of Women's Health, Obstetric and Neonatal Nurses) by Sage Science Press (2455 Teller Road, Thousand Oaks, CA 91320-2218, 800-818-7243, http://jognn.awhonn.org). Features articles about the latest advances in childbearing, infant development, maternal psychology, labor technique, and much more.

The Journal of Practical Nursing. Published quarterly by the National Association for Practical Nurse Education and Service Inc. (PO Box 25647, Alexandria, VA 22313-5647, http://www.napnes.org/journal.htm). Offers feature articles, editorials, educational and scholarship information, and features on licensed practical nurses.

Journal of the American Academy of Nurse Practitioners. Published by Blackwell Publishing (350 Main Street, Malden, MA 02148-5020, 800-835-6770, subscrip@bos.blackwellpublishing.com, http://www.blackwellpublishing.com). The official publication of the Academy, this monthly journal offers peer-reviewed articles on clinical practice, health policy, clinical management, and other issues of interest to nurse practitioners.

Journal of the American Medical Association. Published biweekly by the American Medical Association (PO Box 10946, Chicago, IL 60610-0946,

312-670-7827, ama-subs@ama-assn. org, http://jama.ama-assn.org), this scholarly journal addresses topics in medicine and public health, which are of interest to doctors, scientists, and researchers in related fields. Each issue contains sections with original research studies, medical news and perspectives, book reviews, editorials, and more. The journal is accessible online, but only with a paid subscription.

Journal of the American Physical Therapy Association. Published monthly by the American Physical Therapy Association (1111 North Fairfax Street, Alexandria, VA 22314-1488, 800-999-2782, ext. 3197, ptjourn@apta. org, http://www.ptjournal.org), this scholarly research journal for physical therapists has five sections: research reports, perspectives, updates, letters to the editor, and evidence in practice. Each of the first three sections contains abstracts and full-text articles, available online without a subscription. While technical in nature, individuals researching any particular related physical ailment, or those wanting to learn more about what physical therapy is all about, will find the articles useful.

Medical-Surgical Nursing Journal. Published monthly by Anthony J. Jannetti Inc. (East Holly Avenue, Box 56, Pitman, NJ 08071-0056, 856-256-2300, http://www.ajj.com/services/pblshng/msnj). The official journal of the Academy of Medical-Surgical Nurses, it provides readers with useful, multidis-ciplinary information about providing clinically excellent patient care in various surgical settings.

Midwifery Today Magazine. Published quarterly by Midwifery Today Inc. (PO Box 2672, Eugene, OR 97402-0223, 800-743-0974, inquiries@midwiferyto-day.com, http://www.midwiferytoday. com/magazine). Offers articles about issues that are important to nurse midwives, including multiple births, homebirth, water birth, birth and disability, prenatal and postpartum care, and midwifery education.

Modern Healthcare. Published weekly by Crain Communications (360 North Michigan Avenue, 5th Floor, Chicago IL 60601-3806, 312-649-5350 or 5297, subs@crain.com, http://www.modern-healthcare.com), this timely news publication for business executives in the health care industry provides the most up-to-date, breaking business news in the health care industry. Subscribers can choose to pay extra to receive daily e-mail summaries of health care-related news. Breaking news e-mail alerts are an added benefit subscribers receive.

Nurse Educator. Published bimonthly by Lippincott Williams & Wilkins (PO Box 1620, Hagerstown, MD 21741-1620, 800-638-3030, http://www. nurseeducatoronline.com). Discusses many issues of mentorship and professional role development in undergraduate and graduate nursing education. Offers a sense of what nursing educators look for in their students and peers.

NurseWeek. Published weekly by Nurse-Week Publishing (6860 Santa Teresa Boulevard, San Jose, CA 95119-1205, 800-859-2091, ce@nursingspectrum.com). Offers interesting articles about practice issues for nurses, including job sharing, diversity, pain management, and medical developments. View sample articles at http://www.nurseweek.com/news/features.asp.

Nursing History Review. Published annually by Springer Publishing Company (536 Broadway, New York, NY 10012-9904, 212-431-4370, contactus@springerpub.com, http://www.aahn.org/nhr.html). Official journal of the American Association for the History of Nursing. Contains essays, editorials, articles, and reviews about nursing methods, theories, and movements.

Nursing Spectrum. Published online (http://www.nursingspectrum.com) by Nursing Spectrum. Features a variety of interesting articles written by experienced nurses. Topics include practice issues, nursing careers, jobs, education, certification, and financial aid. Print issues on special topics are also available.

Online Journal of Issues in Nursing. Published by the Kent State University College of Nursing and the American Nurses Association and available for free at http://nursingworld.org/ojin. An excellent forum for discussing and learning about pertinent issues in nursing.

Pediatrics in Review. Published monthly by the American Academy of Pediatrics (141 Northwest Point Boulevard, Elk Grove Village, IL 60007-1098, 866-843-2271, journals@aap.org, http://pedsinreview.aappublications.org), this journal for pediatricians covers the latest news and research findings in the industry as well as provides continuing education support by reviewing topics of importance to industry practitioners. Articles are available by paid subscription only and are primarily intended for individuals with a working knowledge of pediatric medicine.

Plastic Surgical Nursing Journal. Published by the American Society for Plastic Surgical Nurses (7794 Grow Drive, Pensacola, FL 32514-7072, http://www.aspsn.org). Offers information on continuing education, updates on current techniques, and information on new tools and products for plastic surgical nurses.

Practical Nursing Journal. Published quarterly by the National Federation of Licensed Practical Nurses Inc. (605 Poole Drive, Garner, NC 27529-5203, http://www.nflpn.org). Includes articles about professional and personal issues for licensed practical nurses, health industry trends, careers, and continuing education.

RN. Published monthly by Advanstar Communications (Five Paragon Drive Montvale, NJ 07645-1742, 800-284-8945, RNMagazine@advanstar.com, http://www.rnweb.com/rnweb). The content of this publication is geared toward RNs working in hospital-affiliated facilities. Approximately 80 percent of the articles focus on clinical issues. Other subjects that are covered include legal issues, ethical questions, and career development.

The Student Journal of Nurse Anesthesia. Published quarterly by the American Association of Nurse Anesthetists (222 South Prospect Avenue, Park Ridge, IL 60068-4001, http://www.aana.com). Offers case reports and abstracts about nurse anesthesia issues authored by graduate nursing students. It is distributed free of charge to all student members of the association.

Surf the Web

You must use the Internet to do research, to find out, and to explore. Short of an "all health care, all the time" channel on TV, the Internet is the closest you'll get to what's happening now all over the place. This chapter gets you started with an annotated list of Web sites related to health care. Try a few. Follow the links. Maybe even venture as far as asking questions in a chat room. The more you read about health care and interact with professionals in the field, the better prepared you'll be when you're old enough to participate as a professional.

One caveat: you probably already know that URLs change all the time. If a Web address listed below is out of date, try searching the site's name or other key words. Chances are that if it's still out there, you'll find it. If it's not, maybe you'll find something better!

American Association of Colleges of Nurses (AACN)
http://www.aacn.nche.edu

The AACN describes itself as the national voice for nursing education programs, and at first glimpse this site may seem too academic. But delve into the right sections and you'll see that it contains some precious nuggets for students considering a future in nursing. In fact, one of this site's most useful tools is specifically aimed at nurses-to-be. Under a section called Nursing Education, you'll find a lengthy, informative article that debunks some misconceptions about the field and explores the changing job market. There's also a financial aid fact sheet and a directory of AACN's more than 500 member schools.

This extremely well-organized site also includes a schedule of upcoming conferences and seminars. If academics are your thing, go ahead and read AACN's newsletter and other related publications online. The emphasis is on government affairs and college accreditation, topics that will probably be of more interest to the professional nurse.

American Medical Association
http://www.ama-assn.org

With origins dating back to 1847, this prestigious association provides medical students and medical professionals with the most up-to-date access to what is happening in the field of medicine. Medical students and residents will find a drop list of categories of particular interest to them that is easy to locate among the main-menu options at the top of the page. From information on health care careers, to medical licensure, to books and CD-ROMS, to an online database of fellowships and residencies (searchable by specialty, location, or optional criteria), students will find this Web site an invaluable resource. Additional main sections provide information on ongoing advocacy efforts in medicine, headline news, publications, professional resources (legal issues, medical ethics), and much more. Beginning students who have not yet applied to medical school won't find a lot of information tailored to them, but they will benefit nevertheless from reviewing topics of relevance to professionals in the field.

American Red Cross
http://www.redcross.org

The Red Cross offers CPR and first aid courses and other types of training to young people who want to educate themselves and others about various health and safety issues. At its Web site, you'll find information on all of these options and many more. There is also a helpful little feature that allows you to type in your zip code and get contact information for the Red Cross office nearest you, so you can get involved right away.

This site, which is both extensive and easy to use, also gives you an interesting history lesson via its Red Cross Museum, and puts you in touch with other humanitarian organizations that share this organization's commitment to helping others. The American Red Cross has been an integral part of the country's health and safety efforts since 1881—it has a lot to offer you as you explore the field of health care, and its Web site deserves a look.

CyberNurse.com
http://www.cybernurse.com

Founded by two nurses who also shared an interest in the Internet, CyberNurse is a fun site to visit. Not only can you find a list of accredited nursing programs nationwide—with links to many of them—but also find "educational moolah" via state and federal links to nursing loans and grants. Basic information is given regarding NCLEX review and testing, as well as links to job postings and nurse recruiters. Do you want a real view of the world of nursing? Visit the Cyber-Nurse Forum, where nurses dish it out regarding everything from the state of the profession today to the latest nurse joke. Don't forget to check out the history of "capping," complete with photos of early nurse uniforms and caps.

Discover Nursing
http://www.discovernursing.com

Get the who, what, why, and how about nursing from this Web site, which is sponsored by Johnson & Johnson Health Care Systems. Sections are headed as such and are full of useful information—all of which are organized and accessible. In "Who," you can find profiles ranging from students, to nurses with disabilities, to males working in a female-dominated field. Links to specific interest organizations and books are also provided. Are you still seeking a good nursing program, or perhaps unsure of how you will pay for your education? "How" can help you find scholarships or other funding choices, as well as narrow your search for the perfect nursing program. Especially useful is the Web site's listing of programs with available enrollment. Not only is Discover

Nursing a great Web site for students, but second-career nurses and foreign-educated nurses will also find this site useful. Definitely worth a long browse!

ExceptionalNurse.com
http://www.exceptionalnurse.com

This is a clearinghouse of information for nurses who have disabilities. The Web site offers a discussion board, details on scholarships, useful articles, and a wealth of other information that will be of use to disabled nurses.

Genetic Counseling
http://www.ornl.gov/sci/
    techresources/Human_Genome/
    medicine/genecounseling.shtml

Individuals researching health careers with a focus on counseling will find this Web site informative. Providing an overview of what the field of genetic counseling entails—from what a genetic counselor is, where to find information, how to become a genetic counselor, and career opportunities available—this Web site does an exceptional job of directing individuals to related sources of information. Students will especially find the articles, additional resources, and books sections important if they are seriously considering the field. The link in this section called "Graduate Programs in Genetic Counseling" provides links to the 23 accredited genetic counseling programs in the United States. The left-hand side of the Web page provides links to a variety of genetics-related topics, as the Web site it hosted by the Human Genome Project.

HealthWeb: Nursing
http://healthweb.org/browse.
    cfm?subjectid=60

An impressive collaborative effort of the Taubman Medical Library, the School of Nursing at the University of Michigan, and the HealthWeb project, this site is a heavyweight of nursing information.

Under the mantle of Career Resources, you can link to the *Occupational Outlook Handbook* in its entirety, or simply click on the nursing sections already plucked out for you, such as working conditions, employment, training, job outlook, earnings, and related occupations. You might be encouraged to read here that employment of registered nurses is expected to grow rapidly through 2014, with many of the new jobs in home health and hospital outpatient facilities.

In the Discussion Groups section, you'll find information and e-mail addresses for a number of online nursing discussion groups. If there's a particular field of nursing that piques your interest, the specialized discussion groups are a good place to gain insight into the field. The Academic Institutions section has online links to international and U.S. nursing schools. Other pages will link you to nursing school newsletters and journals. If you're the kind of person who believes there's no such thing as too much information, you'll love this site.

How Stuff Works: How Emergency Rooms Work
http://people.howstuffworks.com/
    emergency-room.htm

This site should also be on your short list of Web sites to explore, as it covers how "stuff," as varied and timely as tsunamis to identity theft, works. Complex concepts are carefully broken down and examined, including photos and links to current and past news items about the subject. This particular subsite of How It Works provides information about the inner workings of emergency rooms through detailed descriptions and photographs of emergency rooms, tools of the trade (such as stethoscopes, cardiac monitors, and suture trays), and types of workers, including nurses and physicians. Best yet, the articles are written by emergency room physicians, so you're guaranteed an expert look at this sometimes confusing and scary world of emergency care.

Human Anatomy Online
http://www.innerbody.com/htm/
    body.html

Whether you need a little help in your anatomy class or just want to do some exploring on your own, this site offers an interesting way to explore the systems of the human body. You have your choice of 10 systems: cardiovascular, digestive, endocrine, female reproductive, lymphatic, male reproductive, muscular, nervous, skeletal, and urinary.

Every image in every system features points on which you can click to see the name of a selected body part. Click again for a definition or description of that part. Some animation showing the parts in action is also available. This site is simple and straightforward enough for users with little background in human anatomy.

Imagine
http://www.jhu.edu/~gifted/imagine

Imagine is a bimonthly journal for the go-getter high school student with his or her eye on the future. Its tag line, "Opportunities and resources for academically talented youth," says it all.

If you're always searching for good academic programs, competitions, and internships, this publication can keep you well informed on what's available and when you need to apply. There's an entertaining College Review series in which student contributors evaluate individual colleges and universities and also a Career Options series featuring interviews with professionals.

Along with the current issue, selected portions of back issues can be read online. Previous issues have included articles about the health and medical sciences, as well as general tips on entering academic competitions and choosing summer academic programs. For $30 a year, you can subscribe and get the printed journal delivered to your home—or for free, you can just read selected articles online.

Make a Difference: Discover a Career in Healthcare Management!
http://www.healthmanagementcareers.
    org

Geared to a younger audience of students who have yet to make a decision to enter the field of health care, this Web site provides general information to students, educators, and counselors alike. Students will find career profiles and educational information on the types of degrees and backgrounds necessary to enter select health care fields informative, yet broad and a bit generalized. Links to the U.S. Bureau of Labor Statistics and Job Outlook and Healthcare Management Earnings pages might provide especially useful to students weighing their options for the future. Educators and counselors will find downloadable Powerpoint presentations tailored to high school students and undergraduate students particularly useful. All in all, this Web site serves as a great starting point for aspiring health care managers.

My Future
http://www.myfuture.com

You want to become a health care professional, but perhaps a four-year college just isn't in the cards for you. This colorful site aims to help new high school graduates "jumpstart their lives" with information about alternatives to four-year colleges, such as military opportunities and technical or vocational colleges. In the hefty military career database, you'll find dozens of job descriptions for positions such as nurse, medical care technician, physician assistant, registered nurse, and pharmacist.

While the site is divided into four main sections—Military Opportunities, Money Matters, Beyond High School, and Career Toolbox—most of the useful stuff is in the Career section. In this section, for instance, you can learn about the hottest jobs, how to write strong cover letters, or how to ace that interview. You can also take a career interest quiz to find out if you have a realistic, investigative, artistic, social, enterprising, or conventional work personality.

You'll also find some good info in the Money section. In Living On Your Own, you can learn how to set a budget and live within your means. Or visit the section called Searching for Dollars to get a handle on the financial aid process.

National Student Nurses' Association
http://www.nsna.org

This organization's mission is to represent and mentor nursing students, and its Web site does just that. The Career Center will assist young students as well as older, second-career students via essays such as "Is Nursing For You?" and "Juggling Nursing School and Family." Looking for that first job is made easier with the site's listing of available internships, hospitals, and health care agencies grouped by region or magnet status. The Web site also lists available scholarship information and applications in its Foundation section.

Net Frog: The On-Line Dissection
http://curry.edschool.Virginia.EDU/go/frog

Dissect a frog online? If you've got the amphibian, a scalpel, and an Internet connection, you're ready. With color photographs and downloadable QuickTime movies, this Web site just might conjure up the aroma of formaldehyde.

The site was designed to provide a step-by-step interactive tutorial for use in high school biology classrooms. It can also be used as a preparation tool or as a substitute for an actual laboratory dissection. The complete dissection is divided into Set-Up, Incisions, Organs, and Clean-Up sections. In each section, procedures for dissection are clearly described and presented in photographs.

The creators of this site invite your feedback to make it even better. Anybody interested in anatomy will want to check it out, as will students who are thinking of authoring their own tutorial Web site.

Nurse.com

http://www.nurse.com

This Web site is pretty straightforward and easy to navigate, with the usual nurse forums and discussion boards, the latest news regarding the health care industry, and nursing "lite" first person stories. Check out the Career section—every month it features a profile of a specific type of nursing professional. This is a great way to learn the different specialties available in the nursing industry. Also in the Career section are job profiles of positions currently open. Hospitals nationwide are also detailed. It should be noted that most, if not all, jobs and hospitals featured in this section are part of the Tenet Services Inc. network, which maintains and operates this Web site.

NurseWeek

http://www.nurseweek.com

NurseWeek, an online magazine, operates like a professional clipping service for nurses. At its home page, you can read today's medical and nursing news. Recent headlines, for example, featured a research campaign to prevent premature births, the growing shortage of nursing school instructors, and the benefits of dark chocolate. Continuing education opportunities and career fairs worldwide are also listed.

This is a comprehensive, appealing, and eclectic read for those in the nursing or health care field. One of *NurseWeek*'s regular features is an online survey where you can simply answer "yes" or "no" or submit a full letter to the editor. In subsequent editions of the magazine, readers can see the survey results online. *NurseWeek* also publishes lengthier articles about the nursing profession, and recently, a special career guide for student nurses. Students can also use this site to learn about the job market, as well as create and post their resumes online.

And what Web site would be complete without links to other Web sites? That's right; *NurseWeek* offers many links to other nursing resources—such as education, jobs, and nursing supplies.

Peterson's Planner

http://www.petersons.com

This site offers anything you want to know about surviving high school, getting into college, and choosing a graduate degree. Specific to nursing, check out the College and Graduate School sections, which offer school directories searchable by keyword, degree, location, tuition, size, GPA, and even sports offered. While this site is not devoted solely to health care education, visit it for its comprehensiveness; school listings offer the usual basics plus details on financial aid, school facilities, student government, faculty, and admissions requirements.

The Pfizer Guide To Careers for Physicians
http://www.pfizercareerguides.com/default.asp?t=book&b=physicians

If you're thinking of becoming a physician, this Web site offers an easy-to-read guide that serves as a useful resource as you begin your journey. With well-defined categories and subcategories on the left-hand side of the page, each click takes you to an advice-filled page of practical and meaningful information. "Beginning Your Journey in Medicine," for example, is written in advice-column style by a physician, who points out what she considers important things to remember as you begin medical school. The site stresses the importance of developing mentoring relationships and not giving up the types of volunteer activities that you may have participated in prior to your hectic new med-student life. With sections dedicated to various practice areas, planning your career path, and a complete directory of organizations and additional resources, this Web site provides fundamental information of value to anyone thinking about or currently attending medical school. For those who prefer to read on paper versus the computer, the site offers a free downloadable Portable Document Format (PDF) booklet.

The Pfizer Guide to Careers in Nursing
http://www.pfizercareerguides.com/nursing.html

http://www.pfizercareerguide.com/pdfs/nursing.pdf

Nursing students will definitely be interested in this career guide prepared by the pharmaceutical giant, Pfizer. It starts with a career planning chapter, complete with resume tips and "words of wisdom." The best part of this guide is the "Practice Areas" chapter on 31 nursing specialties. Told through the eyes of a nurse practicing in each specific specialty, you can really get a feel of what it takes, for example, to be an ER nurse, forensic nurse, or a military nurse. Each article ends with a Fast Fact section that details education and certification requirements, necessary skills, and possible employment paths. This guide also devotes a chapter to the Associate Degree of Nursing (ADN), explaining some of the benefits of choosing this shorter educational path, and providing a list of possible practice areas open to nurses holding an ADN.

Be warned that this guide is presented in a Portable Document Format (PDF) and may be a little tedious to navigate.

The Pfizer Guide to Careers in Public Health
http://www.pfizercareerguides.com/publichealth.html

This Web link provides a free, downloadable (in PDF) 33-chapter booklet on careers in public health. You can expect to find first-person accounts of the day-to-day experiences of real public health professionals that will serve as testimonies to this dynamic career field. At 219 pages, this guidebook profiles job titles under subheadings such as Health Policy and Management, Family Health, Occupational Safety, International and Global Health, and many more. Chapters contain additional related articles and essays as well. Finally, a valuable list of universities offering public health degrees concludes the publication.

The Princeton Review
http://www.review.com

This site is everything you want in a high school guidance counselor—it's friendly, well informed, and available to you night and day. Originally a standardized test preparation company, The Princeton Review is now online, giving you frank advice on colleges, careers, and of course, SATs.

Students who've spent their summers and after-school hours volunteering at a clinic or hospital will find good tips here on how to present those extracurricular activities on college application forms. If you're looking for contact with other students who are weighing their options, too, link to one of the discussion groups on college admissions and careers.

Two of the Princeton Review's coolest tools are the Career Quiz, which creates a list of possible careers based on your interests and work style, and the Counselor-O-Matic, which reviews your grades, test scores, and extracurricular record to calculate your chances of admission at many colleges. Also helpful is the list of schools offering online program and degrees. Get a heads-up on the competition by checking out the site's summer program section, specifically geared towards high school students, which lists summer internships, camps, and enrichment programs.

Student Doctor Network
http://www.studentdoctor.net

Whether you've recently begun medical school or are just beginning to think about a career in a health profession, this Web site provides exceptional unbiased support and/or assistance as you take that next big step. Students will especially benefit from the many online forums for premed, dental, podiatry, pharmacy and many more categories and specialties. If you have a question, this is the place to ask as well as to learn from others in the same situation. With tips on what to expect at medical school interviews, how to secure students loans, and writing the application essay, students at varying levels of readiness for a health care career will find this site a useful and valuable resource to learn from others' experience and to share their own.

Tomorrow's Doctors
http://www.aamc.org/students

Sponsored by the Association of American Medical Colleges, this Web site fittingly provides "tomorrow's doctors" with resources galore when it comes to applying to, selecting, and financing medical school. Minority students will find the section called Minorities in Medicine especially useful, with links not only to specialized related organizations, but also to scholarship opportunities. Other sections discuss in great length the options available for financing a medical education—from loan repayment programs to loan forgiveness programs. A wealth of debt management advice is offered. Finally, links to the National Resident Matching Program and ERAS Residency and Osteopathic Internship program provide convenient access to an array of available internships, residencies, and fellowships across the country. Interested candidates can register online and follow the procedures to try to match to a suitable position.

Virtual Family Medicine Interest Group

http://fmignet.aafp.org

This self-proclaimed "family medicine and medical education resource for students" claims it provides relevant information for students throughout their medical educations. With six main categories (family medicine, medical school, residency, clinical resources, leadership/service, and Family Medicine Interest Group on campus), the site is easy to navigate and provides in-depth subcategories in each section. Also of value on this site are the links to the journal publications, *American Family Physician* and *Family Practice Management.* Student membership in the American Academy of Family Physicians is also promoted, as the site is maintained by the Academy. You'll find a shortcut to the membership benefits page in the top upper-left-hand corner.

Ask for Money

By the time most students get around to thinking about applying for scholarships, they have already extolled their personal and academic virtues to such lengths in essays and interviews for college applications that even their own grandmothers wouldn't recognize them. The thought of filling out yet another application form fills students with dread. And why bother? Won't the same five or six kids who have been fighting over grade point averages since the fifth grade walk away with all the really good scholarships?

The truth is, most of the scholarships available to high school and college students are being offered because an organization wants to promote interest in a particular field, encourage more students to become qualified to enter it, and finally, to help those students afford an education. Certainly, having a good grade point average is a valuable asset, and many organizations that grant scholarships request that only applicants with a minimum grade point average apply. More often than not, however, grade point averages aren't even mentioned; the focus is on the area of interest and what a student has done to distinguish himself or herself in that area. In fact, frequently the only requirement is that the scholarship applicant must be studying in a particular area.

❑ GUIDELINES

When applying for scholarships there are a few simple guidelines that can help ease the process considerably.

Plan Ahead

The absolute worst thing you can do is wait until the last minute. For one thing, obtaining recommendations or other supporting data in time to meet an application deadline is incredibly difficult. For another, no one does his or her best thinking or writing under the gun. So get off to a good start by reviewing scholarship applications as early as possible—months, even a year, in advance. If the current scholarship information isn't available, ask for a copy of last year's version. Once you have the scholarship information or application in hand, read it thoroughly. Try to determine how your experience or situation best fits into the scholarship, or even if it fits at all. Don't waste time applying for a scholarship in literature if you couldn't finish *Great Expectations.*

If possible research the award or scholarship, including past recipients and, where applicable, the person in whose name the scholarship is offered. Often, scholarships are general in nature, but some scholarships are meant to memorialize the work of an individual—such as a famous nurse or physician. In those cases, try and get a feel for the spirit of the person's work. If you have any similar interests or experiences, don't hesitate to mention these.

Talk to people who received the scholarship, or to students currently studying in the same area or field of interest in which the scholarship is offered, and try to gain insight into possible applications or work related to that field. The more you know, the more specific you can be when writing your essay explaining why you want this scholarship, for example—"I would benefit from receiving this scholarship because studying geriatric nursing will help me learn about the special needs of the elderly, especially regarding dementia."

Take your time writing the essays. Make certain you are answering the question or questions on the application and not merely restating facts about yourself. Don't be afraid to get creative; try to imagine what you would think of if you had to sift through hundreds of applications—what would you want to know about the candidate? What would convince you that someone was deserving of the scholarship? Work through several drafts and have someone whose advice you respect—a parent, teacher, or guidance counselor—review the essay for grammar and content.

Finally, if you know in advance which scholarships you want to apply for, there might still be time to stack the deck in your favor by getting an internship, volunteering, or working part-time. Bottom line: the more you know about a scholarship and the sooner you learn it, the better.

Follow Directions

Think of it this way—many of the organizations that offer scholarships devote 99.9 percent of their time to something other than the scholarship for which you are applying. Don't pester them for information. Follow the directions on an application, even when asking for additional materials. If the scholarship information specifies that you write for more information, write for it—don't call.

Pay close attention to whether you're applying for an award, a scholarship, a prize, or financial aid. Often these words are used interchangeably, but just as often they have different meanings. An award is usually given for something you have done: built a park or helped distribute meals to the elderly; or something you have created: a design, an essay, a short film, a screenplay, an invention. On the other hand, a scholarship is frequently a renewable sum of money that is given to a person to help defray the costs of college. Scholarships are given to candidates who meet the necessary criteria based on essays, eligibility, or grades, and sometimes all three.

Supply all the necessary documents, information, fees, etc. and make the deadlines. You won't win any scholarships by forgetting to include a recommendation from your history teacher or failing to postmark the application by the deadline. Bottom line: Get it right the first time, on time.

Apply Early

Once you have the application in hand, don't dawdle. If you've requested it far enough in advance, there shouldn't be any reason for you not to turn it in well ahead of the deadline. You never know, if it comes down to two candidates, the deciding factor just might be who was more on the ball. Bottom line: Don't wait, don't hesitate.

Be Yourself

Don't make promises you can't keep. There are plenty of hefty scholarships available, but if they all require you to study something that you don't enjoy, you'll be miserable in college. And the side effects from switching majors after you've accepted a scholarship could be even worse. Bottom line: Be yourself.

Don't Limit Yourself

There are many sources for scholarships, beginning with your guidance counselor and ending with the Internet. All of the search engines have education categories. Start there and search by keywords, such as "financial aid," "scholarship," "award." Don't be limited to the scholarships listed in these pages.

If you know of an organization related to or involved with the field of your choice, write a letter asking if they offer scholarships. If they don't offer scholarships, don't let that stop you. Write them another letter, or better yet, schedule a meeting with the president or someone in the public relations office and ask them if they would be willing to sponsor a scholarship for you. Of course, you'll need to prepare yourself well for such a meeting because you're selling a priceless commodity—yourself. Don't be shy, be confident. Tell them all about yourself, what you want to study and why, and let them know what you would be willing to do in exchange—volunteer at their favorite charity, write up reports on your progress in school, or work part-time on school breaks, full-time, or during the summer. Explain why you're a wise investment.

❏ THE LIST

Air Force ROTC
551 East Maxwell Boulevard
Maxwell AFB, AL 36112-5917
866-423-7682
http://www.afrotc.com

The Air Force ROTC provides a wide range of four-year scholarships (ranging to partial or full tuition) to high school students planning to study health care or other majors in college. Scholarships are also available to college and enlisted students. Visit the Air Force ROTC Web site to apply.

Alpha Tau Delta
Scholarship Chair
11252 Camarillo Street
Toluca Lake, CA 91602
http://www.atdnursing.org

Alpha Tau Delta (ATD) is a national fraternity for professional nurses. Undergraduate and graduate members of an Alpha Tau Delta chapter are eligible for grants to help finance nursing training. Applicants must have strong academic records and demonstrate financial need. Amounts vary; contact ATD for more information.

American Academy of Nurse Practitioners Foundation Scholarship and Grant Program

PO Box 10729
Glendale, AZ 85318-0729
623-376-9467
foundation@aanp.org
http://www.aanpfoundation.org

The foundation offers a variety of scholarships and grants to undergraduate and graduate nurse practitioner students. Contact the foundation for more information.

American Academy of Orthotists and Prosthetists

Orthotic and Prosthetic Education and Development Fund
526 King Street, Suite 201
Alexandria, VA 22314
703-836-0788, ext. 206
scholarship@oandp.org
http://www.oandp.org/education

The academy offers several scholarships to students pursuing study in accredited orthotics and prosthetics bachelor's degree programs. Visit the academy's Web site to download applications.

American Assembly for Men in Nursing Foundation

PO Box 130220
Birmingham, AL 35213
205-802-7551
http://www.aamn.org/
    aamnfoundationscholarships.htm

The assembly offers scholarships to male nursing students as funds are available.

Visit the foundation's Web site for more information.

American Association of Colleges of Nursing (AACN)

CampusRN/AACN Scholarship Fund
One Dupont Circle, NW, Suite 530
Washington, DC 20036
202-463-6930
http://www.aacn.nche.edu/
    Education/financialaid.htm

The association awards six $2,500 scholarships to students who are seeking baccalaureate, master's, or doctoral degrees in nursing. Preference will be given to students who are enrolled in a master's or doctoral program and plan to pursue a nursing faculty career; completing an RN-to-baccalaureate program; or enrolled in an accelerated baccalaureate or master's degree nursing program. Contact the AACN for more information.

American Association of Critical-Care Nurses (AACN)

Attn: Scholarships
101 Columbia
Aliso Viejo, CA 92656-4109
800-899-2226
info@aacn.org
http://www.aacn.org/AACN/Memship.
    nsf/vwdoc/mainawards

Educational Advancement Scholarships of $1,500 annually are open to current members or those enrolled full- or part-time in a nursing education program. Applicants must be in their junior year of college and have at least one year of experience working in a critical-care unit. Twenty percent of the awards will be allocated to qualified ethnic minority applicants. Visit the association's Web site for more information and to apply online.

American Association of Neuroscience Nurses

Neuroscience Nursing Foundation
4700 West Lake Avenue
Glenview, IL 60025
888-557-2266
info@aann.org
http://www.aann.org/nnf

The foundation offers a $1,500 annual award to registered nurses who are pursuing studies to advance a career in neuroscience nursing at the undergraduate or graduate level. Contact the foundation for more information.

American Association of Nurse Anesthetists (AANA) Foundation

Student Scholarship Application
222 South Prospect Avenue
Park Ridge, IL 60068-4001
http://www.aana.com/Default.aspx

Students who are currently studying to become nurse anesthetists at an accredited program can apply for a variety of scholarships ranging from $1,000 to $5,000 from the foundation and affiliated organizations. Applicants must be AANA members and have completed a specific level of coursework depending on their grade level. Visit the "Professional Development" section of the foundation's Web site for more information.

American Holistic Nurses' Association (AHNA)

PO Box 2130
Flagstaff, AZ 86003-2130
800-278-2462
info@ahna.org
http://www.ahna.org/edu/assist.html

The Charlotte McGuire Scholarship is offered to nurses undertaking a holistic nursing program; applicants must be members of the AHNA for at least six months and have a minimum 3.0 GPA. The amount of the award varies; contact the association for more information.

American Horticultural Therapy Association (AHTA)

3570 East 12th Avenue, Suite 206
Denver, CO 80206
303-322-2482, 800-634-1603
http://www.ahta.org/grantsAwards/awards.html

Applicants for the Ann Lane Mavromatis Scholarship should have a declared major in the field of horticultural therapy or a related field with course work supporting the field of horticultural therapy, membership in the AHTA, a high level of academic achievement, evidence of financial need, and personal involvement in horticultural therapy through contribution to the development of the horticultural therapy program at their college or university or through participation in extracurricular horticultural therapy activities with a local, state, or national horticultural therapy organization. The scholarship is also available to graduate students. Contact the association for more information.

American Indian Science and Engineering Society (AISES)

PO Box 9828
Albuquerque, NM 87119-9828
505-765-1052
http://www.aises.org/highered/
    scholarships

The AISES offers the A.T. Anderson Memorial Scholarship Native American students at the undergraduate or graduate level pursuing study in the sciences, engineering, medicine, natural resources, and mathematics. Contact the society for more information and to download applications.

American Legion Auxiliary

777 North Meridian Street, Third
    Floor
Indianapolis, IN 46204-1420
317-955-3845
alahq@legion-aux.org
http://www.legion-aux.org

Various state auxiliaries of the American Legion offer scholarships to help students prepare for health care and other careers. Most require that candidates be associated with the organization in some way, whether as a child, spouse, etc., of a military veteran. Interested students should contact the auxiliary for further information.

American Alliance for Health, Physical Education, Recreation and Dance (AAHPERD)

Attn: Deb Callis
1900 Association Drive
Reston, VA 20191-1598
708-476-3400, 800-213-7193
dcallis@aahperd.org
http://www.aahperd.org/aahperd/
    template.cfm?template=presidents_
    scholarships.html

Applicants for the Ruth Abernathy Undergraduate Scholarship must be current members of AAHPERD (or join at time of application) who are majoring in the field of health, physical education, recreation, or dance. They must also be full-time students with a junior or senior status at a baccalaureate-granting college or university, maintain a 3.5 out of 4.0 GPA, demonstrate exceptional leadership abilities, and participate in community service activities. Graduate students may also apply for this scholarship. Visit the alliance's Web site to download an application.

American Health Information Management Association (AHIMA) Foundation of Research and Education

233 North Michigan Avenue,
    Suite 2150
Chicago, IL 60601
312-233-1131
http://www.ahima.org/fore/

Applicants for the Merit Scholarship must have at least one full semester of classes remaining in their course of study at the time the award is granted. They also must be members of AHIMA, maintain a minimum 3.0 GPA, and demonstrate a commitment to volunteerism and the health information management profession. The scholarship is also available to graduate students. Contact the foundation for more information.

American Medical Technologists
710 Higgins Road
Park Ridge, IL 60068
800-275-1268
http://www.amt1.com/site/
   epage/9664_315.htm

Applicants for the American Medical Technologists Student Scholarship must be pursuing a course of study that leads to a career in one of the disciplines certified by American Medical Technologists. Applicants must also provide evidence of financial need or career goals. High school seniors may apply. The scholarship is also available to recent graduates of postsecondary programs and medical technologists who are interested in continuing their education. Visit the organization's Web site for more information.

American Psychiatric Nurses Association
1555 Wilson Boulevard, Suite 515
Arlington, VA 22209
703-243-2443
inform@apna.org
http://www.apna.org/foundation/
   scholarships.html

The association offers scholarships to students who are currently studying psychiatric nursing. Visit its Web site for more information.

American School Health Association
Attn: Pamela Dean
7263 State Route 43
Kent, OH 44240
330-678-1601

pdean@ashaweb.org
http://www.ashaweb.org

Applicants for the American School Health Association Scholarship must be college juniors or seniors and graduate students enrolled full-time at an institute of higher education and maintain at least a 3.0 GPA. They also must have declared a major in school health education, school nursing, or pediatric or adolescent medicine or dentistry. Applicants with other school health specializations will be considered only if accompanied by a letter form the applicant's academic advisor stating the program's relationship to school health.

American Society for Clinical Laboratory Science
Attn: Joe Briden, Scholarship
   Coordinator
7809 South 21st Drive
Phoenix, AZ 85041-7736
301-657-2768
http://www.ascls.org/leadership/
   awards/amt.asp

The society offers several scholarships to college juniors and seniors who are attending a National Accrediting Agency for Clinical Laboratory Sciences-accredited undergraduate clinical laboratory science program. They must be in their last year of study when the scholarship is awarded. Visit the society's Web site for more information.

American Society of Radiologic Technologists (ASRT) Education and Research Foundation
Scholarship Program

15000 Central Avenue, SE
Albuquerque, NM 87123
800-444-2778, ext. 2541
foundation@asrt.org
http://www.asrt.org/
    content/ASRTFoundation/
    AwardsandScholarships/Awards_
    Scholarships.aspx

The society offers several scholarships for students pursuing entry-level study in the radiological sciences, as well as professionals who are interested in continuing their education. Visit the society's Web site for more information.

Army ROTC
800-USA-ROTC
http://www.goarmy.com/rotc/
    scholarships.jsp

Students planning to or currently pursuing a bachelor's degree may apply for scholarships that pay tuition and some living expenses; recipients must agree to accept a commission and serve in the Army on Active Duty or in a Reserve Component (U.S. Army Reserve or Army National Guard).

Association of periOperative Registered Nurses (AORN)
2170 South Parker Road, Suite 300
Denver, CO 80231-5711
800-755-2676, ext. 328
ibendzsa@aorn.org
http://www.aorn.org/foundation/
    scholarships.asp

Undergraduate, graduate, and doctoral students who are active or associate members of the association are eligible for scholarships covering tuition and fees. Guidelines vary by scholarship; contact the AORN for further details.

Association of Surgical Technologists (AST)
AST Continuing Education
    Department
6 West Dry Creek Circle
Littleton, CO 80120
800-637-7433
Kfrey@ast.org
http://www.ast.org/Content/
    Education/Scholarships.htm

The association offers several scholarships for students pursuing study in surgical technology. Visit its Web site for more information.

Association of University Programs in Health Administration
2000 North 14th Street, Suite 780
Arlington, VA 22201
703-894-0940
aupha@aupha.org
http://www.aupha.org

The association offers scholarships and fellowships to graduate students who are pursuing study in health care administration. Visit the association's Web site for more information.

Association on American Indian Affairs
Scholarship Coordinator
966 Hungerford Drive, Suite 12-B
Rockville, MD 20850
240-314-7155
general.aaia@verizon.net
http://www.indian-affairs.org

Undergraduate and graduate Native American students who are pursuing a wide variety of college majors (including nursing and other health care fields) can apply for several different scholarships ranging from $500 to $1,500. All applicants must provide proof of Native American heritage. Visit the association's Web site for more information.

Business and Professional Women's Foundation

1900 M Street, NW, Suite 310
Washington, DC 20036
202-293-1100
http://www.bpwusa.org

The foundation's Career Advancement Scholarship Program awards scholarships to women in health-related professions. Applicants must be at least 25 years old, accepted by or attending an accredited university program, plan to graduate within 12 to 24 months of the awarding of the grant, demonstrate financial need, and be U.S. citizens. Visit the foundation's Web site for deadlines and to download an application.

Chi Eta Phi Sorority Inc.

3029 13th Street, NW
Washington, DC 20009
202-232-3858
chietaphi@erols.com
http://www.chietaphi.com/scholar.html

The sorority offers scholarships to minority students currently enrolled in a program of study leading to the baccalaureate, master's, or doctoral degree in an accredited school of nursing. Visit its Web site for further details.

Collegeboard.com

http://apps.collegeboard.com/
    cbsearch_ss/welcome.jsp

This testing service (PSAT, SAT, etc.) also offers a scholarship search engine at its Web site. It features scholarships (not all health care-related) worth more than $3 billion. You can search by specific majority and a variety of other criteria.

CollegeNET

http://mach25.collegenet.com/cgi-bin/
    M25/index

CollegeNET features 600,000 scholarships (not all broadcasting-related) worth more than $1.6 billion. You can search by keyword (such as "health care" and "nursing") or by creating a personality profile of your interests.

Daughters of the American Revolution (DAR)

Scholarship Committee
1776 D Street, NW
Washington, DC 20006-5303
202-628-1776
http://www.dar.org

DAR offers a variety of scholarships to students interested in pursuing careers in health care. Caroline Holt Nursing Scholarships are available to students who have been accepted or who are currently enrolled in a nursing program in the United States. Selection criteria include academic standing, financial need, and letters of recommendation; applicants need not be affiliated with DAR. The Mildred Nutting Nursing Scholarship is also available; preference for this scholarships will be given to candidates from the greater Lowell, Massachusetts, area. The Madeline Pickett (Halbert) Cogswell Nursing Scholarship is available to students who are members, descendents of members, or eligible for membership in the DAR and who are accepted or enrolled in an accredited school of nursing. The Occupational/ Physical Therapy Scholarship is available to students who demonstrate financial need and who are attending an accredited school of art, music, occupational, or physical therapy. Students who have been accepted into college or are studying to become a medical doctor (not pre-med) may apply for the Irene and Daisy MacGregor Memorial Scholarship and the Alice W. Rooke Scholarship. Students who are pursuing graduate-level study in psychiatric nursing may also apply for the Daisy MacGregor Memorial Scholarship. Contact DAR for more information.

Discover Nursing
http://www.discovernursing.com/
  scholarship_search.aspx

This Web site, sponsored by Johnson & Johnson, offers a nursing scholarship search engine (as well as extensive career information). You can search by scholarship by keyword, state GPA, ethnicity, and grade level.

Emergency Nurses Association
915 Lee Street
Des Plaines, IL 60016-6569
800-900-9659, ext. 4100
foundation@ena.org
http://www.ena.org/foundation/
  grants

The association offers scholarships ranging from $2,000 to $10,000 to undergraduate and graduate students who are currently enrolled in nursing programs. Visit its Web site to download an application.

ExceptionalNurse.com
Scholarship Committee
13019 Coastal Circle
Palm Beach Gardens, FL 33410
http://www.exceptionalnurse.com/
  scholarship.html

Nursing students with disabilities may apply for scholarships of $250 or $500. Preference is given to undergraduates. Visit ExceptionalNurse.com to download an application.

FastWeb
Web: http://fastweb.monster.com

FastWeb is one of the largest scholarship search engines around. It features 600,000 scholarships (not all health care-related) worth more than $1 billion. To use this resource, you will need to register (free).

Foundation for the Carolinas
PO Box 34769
Charlotte, NC 28234
704-973-4500
infor@fftc.org
http://www.fftc.org

The foundation administers more than 70 scholarship funds that offer awards to undergraduate and graduate students pursuing study in nursing, dental medicine, and other disciplines. Visit its Web site for a searchable list of awards.

Golden Key International Honor Society
621 North Avenue, NE, Suite C-100
Atlanta , GA 30308
800-377-2401
http://www.goldenkey.org

Golden Key is an academic honor society that offers its members "opportunities for individual growth through leadership, career development, networking, and service." It awards more than $400,000 in scholarships annually through 17 different award programs. Membership in the society is selective; only the top 15 percent of college juniors and seniors—who may be pursuing education in any college major—are considered for membership by the organization. There is a one-time membership fee of $60 to $65. Contact the society for more information.

GuaranteedScholarships.com
http://www.guaranteed-scholarships.com

This Web site offers lists (by college) of scholarships, grants, and financial aid (not all health care-related) that "require no interview, essay, portfolio, audition, competition, or other secondary requirement."

Hawaii Community Foundation
1164 Bishop Street, Suite 800
Honolulu, HI 96813
scholarships@hcf-hawaii.org
http://www.
    hawaiicommunityfoundation.org/
    scholar/scholar.php

The foundation offers a variety of scholarships for high school seniors and college students planning to or currently studying health and other majors in college. Applicants must be residents of Hawaii, demonstrate financial need, and plan to attend a two- or four-year college. Visit the foundation's Web site for more information and to apply online.

Health Occupations Students of America (HOSA)
6021 Morriss Road, Suite 111
Flower Mound, TX 75028
800-321-HOSA
http://www.hosa.org

HOSA works with schools "to promote career opportunities in the health care industry and to enhance the delivery of quality health care to all people." It teams with the following organizations to offer more than $40,000 in scholarships to students interested in health care careers: Delmar, Hobsons, Hospital Corporation of America, Kaiser Permanente Healthcare, National Honor Roll, National Technical Honor Society, Nursing Spectrum, and Who's Who Among American High School Students. Contact HOSA for more information.

Health Resources and Services Administration (HRSA)
U.S. Department of Health and
    Human Services
Nursing Scholarship Program
Parklawn Building
5600 Fishers Lane
Rockville, MD 20857
http://bhpr.hrsa.gov/nursing/
    scholarship

The HRSA's Nursing Scholarship Program pays tuition, required fees, reasonable costs, and a monthly stipend to applicants who are willing, upon graduation, to serve two years at a health care facility that has a critical shortage of nurses. Applicants must be U.S. citizens or nationals and be accepted or enrolled as full- or part-time students in an accredited school of nursing in a professional registered nurse program (baccalaureate, graduate, associate degree, or diploma). Registered nurses preparing for teaching careers also are eligible for scholarships toward graduate study. Apply through the attending institution. Contact the HRSA for more information.

Illinois Career Resource Network

http://www.ilworkinfo.com/icrn.htm

Created by the Illinois Department of Employment Security, this useful site offers a scholarship search engine, as well as detailed information on careers (including those in health care). You can search for health care scholarships based on specialty. This site is available to everyone, not just Illinois residents; you can get a password by simply visiting the site. The Illinois Career Information System is just one example of sites created by state departments of employment security (or departments of labor) to assist students with financial- and career-related issues. After checking out this site, visit your state's department of labor Web site to see what they offer.

International Order of the King's Daughters and Sons

Health Careers Scholarship Department
PO Box 1017
Chautauqua, NY 14722-1017
716-357-4951
http://www.iokds.org

Health Careers Scholarships of up to $1,000 are awarded to students who have completed at least one year of study in nursing, medicine, dentistry, pharmacy, physical or occupational therapy, and medical technologies. Applicants must be U.S. or Canadian citizens and enrolled full time in an accredited institution. Contact the order for deadlines and more information.

John D. Archbold Memorial Hospital

Education and Training Department
PO Box 1018
Thomasville, GA 31799-1018
229-228-2795
http://www.archbold.org/AboutUs/scholarships.htm

Scholarships are available to students who are planning to or currently studying nursing, physical therapy, or another health field; recipients must agree to work for up to three years at the hospital following graduation. Contact the hospital's Education and Training Department for more information.

March of Dimes

Office of Fellowships and Awards
1275 Mamaroneck Avenue
White Plains, NY 10605

202-659-1800
profedu@marchofdimes.com
http://www.marchofdimes.com

Registered nurses who are enrolled in graduate programs of maternal-child nursing are eligible to apply for several $5,000 scholarships. Visit the organization's Web site to learn more and to download an application.

Marine Corps Scholarship Foundation

PO Box 3008
Princeton, NJ 08543-3008
800-292-7777
mcsf@marine-scholars.org
http://www.mcsf.org/site/
    c.ivKVLaMTIuG/b.1677655/k.BEA8/
    Home.htm

The foundation helps children of marines and former marines with scholarships of up to $5,000 for study in nursing and other health fields. To be eligible, you must be a high school graduate or registered as an undergraduate student at an accredited college or vocational/technical institute. Additionally, your total family gross income may not exceed $63,000. Contact the foundation for further details.

Maryland Higher Education Commission

Maryland State Nursing Scholarship
839 Bestgate Road, Suite 400
Annapolis, MD 21401
800-974-0203
http://www.mhec.state.md.us/
    financialAid/ProgramDescriptions/
    prog_nurse.asp

High school seniors and undergraduate and graduate students who are Maryland residents and planning to or currently pursuing nursing education, can apply for $3,000 Maryland State Nursing Scholarships. Applicants must have a GPA of at least 3.0, enroll or be enrolled at a two-year or four-year Maryland college or university, and agree to serve as a full-time nurse in an eligible Maryland health care organization one year for each year of aid received. Visit the Commission's Web site to download an application.

National Alaska Native American Indian Nurses Association (NANAINA)

Attn: Dr. Better Keltner, NANAINA
    Treasurer
3700 Reservoir Road, NW
Washington, DC 20057-1107
888-566-8773
http://www.nanainanurses.org/Main_
    Pages/scholarships.html

Undergraduate and graduate students who are currently enrolled in a nursing program are eligible to apply for Merit Awards of $750. Applicants must be enrolled in a U.S. federally or state-recognized tribe, members of the NANAINA, and full-time students. Visit the association's Web site to download an application.

National Association of Hispanic Nurses (NAHN)

NAHN Awards and Scholarship
    Committee Chair
1501 16th Street, NW

Washington, DC 20036
202-387-2477
info@thehispanicnurses.org
http://thehispanicnurses.org/index.
    php?option=com_content&task=se
    ction&id=28&Itemid=611

Hispanic nursing students who are currently enrolled in a nursing program may apply for scholarships. Applicants must be members of the association, have a GPA of at least 3.0, demonstrate financial need, and show potential for leadership in nursing. Visit the NAHN's Web site to download an application.

National Association of School Nurses (NASN)

1416 Park Street
Castle Rock, CO 80109
303-663-2329
http://www.nasn.org/Default.
    aspx?tabid=71

The association awards scholarships to members who are registered nurses who are interested in pursuing education beyond a bachelor's degree. Visit its Web site to download an application.

National Association of Science Writers

PO Box 890
Hedgesville, WV 25427
304-754-5077
info@nasw.org
http://www.nasw.org

Science writers under the age of 30 can compete in a scholarship award competition. Contact the association for more information.

National Black Nurses Association (NBNA)

8630 Fenton Street, Suite 330
Silver Spring, MD 20910-3803
800-575-6298
http://www.nbna.org/scholarship.htm

The association offers a variety of scholarships ranging from $500 to $2,000 to students who are currently enrolled in nursing programs. Applicants must be members of the NBNA. Visit the association's Web site for further details and to download an application.

National Federation of the Blind

Scholarship Committee
805 Fifth Avenue
Grinnell, IA 50112
641-236-3366
http://www.nfb.org/nfb/default.
    asp?SnID=2127883162

Scholarships are available to blind high school seniors and undergraduates who are interested in or currently studying medicine or general studies. Contact the federation for further details. Visit the federation's Web site for an application.

National Gerontological Nursing Association

7794 Grow Drive
Pensacola, FL 32514
800-723-0560
ngna@puetzamc.com
http://www.ngna.org/all.
    php?l=resources&x=9

Applicants for the Mary Opal Wolanin Undergraduate Scholarship must be enrolled full- or part-time in a nationally accredited U.S. school of nursing and maintain at least a 3.0 GPA. They also must intend to work in a gerontology/geriatric setting after graduation. Visit the association's Web site to download an application.

National Health Service Corps
Scholarship Coordinator
5600 Fishers Lane
Rockville, MD 20857
http://nhsc.bhpr.hrsa.gov/join_us/
  scholarships.asp

National Health Service Corps Scholarships paying tuition and a monthly stipend are available for students training at the graduate level to become family nurse practitioners and nurse-midwives. Recipients must practice one year in an underserved area for each year of aid received. To request an application, call 800-221-9393. Scholarships for other health specialties—such as physicians, physician assistants, and dentists—are also available.

National Student Nurses'
Association Foundation
45 Main Street, Suite 606
Brooklyn, NY 11201
718-210-0705
nsna@nsna.org
http://www.nsna.org

Promise of Nursing Scholarships are available to nursing students in selected regions. Visit the foundation's Web site for more information and to download scholarship applications.

Navy: Careers: Healthcare
http://www.navy.com/healthcare

The Navy provides financial support for students interested in studying to become physicians, dentists, nurses, and other types of medical professionals; recipients must later serve on active duty with the Navy. Contact your local recruiter for details.

Oncology Nursing Society
Foundation
125 Enterprise Drive
RIDC Park West
Pittsburgh, PA 15275-1214
412-859-6100
foundation@ons.org
http://onsfoundation.org

Registered nurses enrolled in an undergraduate or graduate program who are interested in oncology nursing may apply for $2,000, $3,000, and $5,000 scholarships. Contact the foundation for further information.

Pedorthic Footwear Foundation
7150 Columbia Gateway Drive,
  Suite G
Columbia, MD 21046
info@pedorthics.org
http://www.pedorthics.org/pages.
  cfm?page=scholarship.html

The Pedorthic Footwear Foundation Scholarship for Pedorthic Education is open to undergraduates studying orthotics and prosthetics pedorthics or podiatry. Applicants must be at least 18 years old and have at least a high school diploma or equivalent. They must have prior experience related to footwear or foot care. Applicants are expected to sit for the certification exam within two years of completing course work supported by the foundation scholarship. The scholarship is also available to medical students. Applicants must submit a completed application and three letters of recommendation. Visit the foundation's Web site to download an application. Deadline: January 15.

Pilot International Foundation
PO Box 4844
Macon, GA 31208-4844
478-743-7403
pifinfo@pilothq.org
http://www.pilotinternational.org/
   html/foundation/scholar.shtml

Undergraduate students preparing for careers working with people with disabilities or brain-related disorders are eligible for scholarships; applicants must be members of a local Pilot Club. Contact the foundation for details.

Sallie Mae
http://www.collegeanswer.com

This Web site offers a scholarship database of more than 2.4 million awards (not all health care-related) worth more than $14 billion. You must register (free) to use the database.

Scholarship America
One Scholarship Way
St. Peter, MN 56082
800-537-4180
http://www.scholarshipamerica.org

This organization works through its local Dollars for Scholars chapters in 41 states and the District of Columbia. In 2003, it awarded more than $29 million in scholarships to students. Visit Scholarship America's Web site for more information.

Scholarships.com
http://www.scholarships.com

Scholarships.com offers a free college scholarship search engine (although you must register to use it) and financial aid information.

Society of Diagnostic Medical Sonography (SDMS) Educational Foundation
2745 Dallas Parkway, Suite 350
Plano, TX 75093-8730
800-229-9506
http://www.sdms.org/foundation/
   scholarships.asp

The SDMS Educational Foundation offers scholarships to students who demonstrate financial need, have high academic achievement, and pursue study in sonography. Visit the society's Web site for details.

United Negro College Fund (UNCF)
http://www.uncf.org/scholarships

Visitors to the UNCF Web site can search for thousands of scholarships and grants, many of which are administered by the UNCF. High school seniors and undergraduate and graduate students who are interested in health care and other careers are eligible. The search engine allows you to search by state, scholarship title, grade level, and achievement score.

U.S. Public Health Service
Division of Health Professions
    Support
Indian Health Service Scholarship
    Program (IHSSP)
801 Thompson Avenue, Suite 120
Rockville, MD 20852
 301-443-6197
bmiller@na.ihs.gov
http://www.ihs.gov/JobsCareerDevelop/
    DHPS/Scholarships/Scholarship_
    index.asp

The Health Professions Preparatory Scholarship Program provides awards to Native American students who are preparing for entry into more than 25 health care fields. Recipients must serve one year in an Indian health facility for each year of aid received. Visit the IHSSP's Web site for more information.

Look to the Pros

The following professional organizations offer a variety of materials, from career brochures to lists of accredited schools to salary surveys. Many of them also publish journals and newsletters that you should become familiar with. Many also have annual conferences that you might be able to attend. (While you may not be able to attend a conference as a participant, it may be possible to "cover" one for your school or even your local paper, especially if your school has a related club.)

When contacting professional organizations, keep in mind that they all exist primarily to serve their members, be it through continuing education, professional licensure, political lobbying, or just "keeping up with the profession." While many are strongly interested in promoting their profession and passing information about it to the general public, these busy professional organizations are not there solely to provide you with information. Whether you call or write, be courteous, brief, and to the point. Know what you need and ask for it. If the organization has a Web site, check it out first: what you're looking for may be available there for downloading, or you may find a list of prices or instructions, such as sending a self-addressed, stamped envelope with your request. Finally, be aware that organizations, like people, move. To save time when writing, first confirm the address, preferably with a quick phone call to the organization itself, "Hello, I'm calling to confirm your address…"

❏ THE SOURCES

Alpha Tau Delta
Scholarship Chair
11252 Camarillo Street
Toluca Lake, CA 91602-1259
http://www.atdnursing.org

Alpha Tau Delta is a national fraternity for professional nurses. It offers financial aid to its members, as well as a nursing job search engine at its Web site.

American Academy of Allergy, Asthma, and Immunology
555 East Wells Street, Suite 1100
Milwaukee, WI 53202-3823
414-272-6071
info@aaaai.org
http://www.aaaai.org

The academy offers career information, a list of accredited training programs, and other resources at its Web site.

American Academy of Dermatology (AAD)
PO Box 4014
Schaumburg, IL 60168-4014

888-503-7546
http://www.aad.org

The AAD can give you good medical information on dermatological conditions as well as employment opportunities and professional concerns.

American Academy of Family Physicians (AAFP)

PO Box 11210
Shawnee Mission, KS 66207-1210
800-274-2237
fp@aafp.org
http://www.aafp.org

Visit the AAFP Web site to access career information, including the virtual family interest group where medical students and residents can find links to career Web sites and loan forgiveness programs. Reduced AAFP membership dues are available for medical students and residents.

American Academy of Nurse Practitioners (AANP)

PO Box 12846
Austin, TX 78711-2846
512-442-4262
admin@aanp.org
http://www.aanp.org

The AANP offers information on national certification, scholarships, professional competencies, membership for nursing students, employment opportunities, and a searchable database of nurse practitioner programs in the United States and throughout the world. You can also visit its Web site to read *A Nurse Practitioner is Your Partner in Health*.

American Academy of Pediatrics

141 Northwest Point Boulevard
Elk Grove Village, IL 60007-1098
847-434-4000
http://www.aap.org

Visit the academy's Web site for an overview of pediatric health issues and to read *Pediatrics 101*, a useful career publication.

American Assembly for Men in Nursing

PO Box 130220
Birmingham, AL 35213-0220
205-802-7551
aamn@aamn.org
http://www.aamn.org

The assembly is a support organization for male nurses. It offers scholarships, an online discussion forum, and membership to male and female nurses, nursing students, and the general public.

American Association of Colleges of Nursing

One Dupont Circle, NW, Suite 530
Washington, DC 20036-1135
202-463-6930
http://www.aacn.nche.edu

The association offers information for nursing students and educators, including a nurse educator career summary, online courses, job listings, information on scholarships for currently enrolled nursing students, and online publications for nurses, such as *Your Nursing Career: A Look at the Facts and What Nursing Grads Should Consider When Seeking Employment*.

American Association of Critical-Care Nurses

101 Columbia
Aliso Viejo, CA 92656-4109
800-899-2226
info@aacn.org
http://www.aacn.org

This organization offers information on certification, job listings, and professional and consumer (non-nurses who are interested in the field of critical care nursing) membership. It also offers the following useful career publications at its Web site: *About Critical Care Nursing, Areas of Expertise,* and *Tap Into a Career in Critical Care Nursing.*

American Association of Legal Nurse Consultants

401 North Michigan Avenue
Chicago, IL 60611-4255
877-402-2562
info@aalnc.org
http://www.aalnc.org

The association offers information on careers (via online publications such as *What is a LNC?* and *Getting Started in Legal Nurse Consulting*) and certification. It also offers publications, books, and an annual conference.

American Association of Neuroscience Nurses

4700 West Lake Avenue
   Glenview, IL 60025-1468
   888-557-2266
info@aann.org
http://www.aann.org

The association provides information on certification, scholarships, and employment opportunities at its Web site.

American Association of Nurse Anesthetists (AANA)

222 South Prospect Avenue
Park Ridge, IL 60068-4001
847-692-7050
info@aana.com
http://www.aana.com

The AANA offers a variety of useful career information in the Students section of its Web site, including *Questions and Answers about a Career in Nurse Anesthesia*, which answers the most frequently asked questions about the profession. Its Web site also includes information on the history of nurse anesthetist practice, accredited programs, jobs, scholarships, and the qualifications and scope of practice of nurse anesthetists. Students may also be interested in learning more about AANA-sponsored writing contests and its Anesthesia College Bowl.

American Association of Occupational Health Nurses

2920 Brandywine Road, Suite 100
Atlanta, GA 30341-5539
770-455-7757
aaohn@aaohn.org
http://www.aaohn.org

Visit the association's Web site to read an occupational and environmental health nursing profession fact sheet.

American Board of Genetic Counseling

9650 Rockville Pike
Bethesda, MD 20814-3998
301-634-7316
http://www.abgc.net

Visit the board's Web site for information on how and when to apply for certification as well as a listing of accredited graduate schools in the United States and Canada.

American College of Health Care Administrators (ACHCA)

300 North Lee Street, Suite 301
Alexandria, VA 22314-2807
888-88-ACHCA
http://www.achca.org

For information on state licensing, certification, and college student membership, visit the ACHCA's Web site. College students can discover how to start their own campus chapter if one does not already exist.

American College of Healthcare Executives

One North Franklin Street, Suite 1700
Chicago, IL 60606-3424
312-424-2800
GenInfo@ache.org
http://www.ache.org

College students should visit this organization's Web site to learn more about student membership and its benefits. The Education and Career sections contain educational seminar registration sections as well as resume and job banks.

American College of Nurse-Midwives (ACNM)

8403 Colesville Road, Suite 1550
Silver Spring, MD 20910-6374
240-485-1800
http://www.acnm.org

Visit the ACNM's Web site to read *A Career in Midwifery,* which presents a basic overview of the field, educational requirements, and sources of financial aid. Its Web site includes lists of education programs and information on core competencies, financial aid, credentialing and licensure, history and philosophy of nurse-midwifery, and FAQs for students.

American College of Obstetricians and Gynecologists

409 12th Street, SW, PO Box 96920
Washington, DC 20090-6920
202-638-5577
http://www.acog.org

Contact the college for information on obstetrics and gynecology, useful publications, and student (medical) membership.

American Holistic Health Association

PO Box 17400
Anaheim, CA 92817-7400
714-779-6152
mail@ahha.org
http://ahha.org

Visit the association's Web site to read articles on holistic health and access a searchable database of practitioner members. Membership is also available for those interested in holistic health and practitioners.

American Holistic Medical Association

12101 Menaul Boulevard, NE, Suite C
Albuquerque, NM 87112-2460

505-292-7788
ksummers@holisticmedicine.org
http://www.holisticmedicine.org

Visit the association's Web site to learn more about holistic medicine, a searchable database of members, student (college) membership, and to read back issues of the *AHMA Newsletter*.

American Holistic Nurses Association

PO Box 2130
Flagstaff, AZ 86003-2130
800-278-2462
info@ahna.org
http://www.ahna.org

The association provides information on careers in holistic nursing, educational programs, scholarships, and certification at its Web site.

American Hospital Association

One North Franklin
Chicago, IL 60606-3421
312-422-3000
http://www.aha.org

Contact the association for information on hospital-based health care careers.

American Institute of Ultrasound in Medicine

14750 Sweitzer Lane, Suite 100
Laurel, MD 20707-5906
301-498-4100
http://www.aium.org

This organization provides scholarship opportunities for students attending ultrasound programs as well as student memberships. Visit the organization's

Web site for a complete list of membership benefits, including publications, and to view a job board.

American Medical Association

515 North State Street
Chicago, IL 60610-5453
800-621-8335
http://www.ama-assn.org

High school students or early college students will benefit from the Choosing a Health Care Career link, while medical students should visit the site to use the fellowship and resident database, learn about medical licensure, and obtain information about scholarships available to medical students. Student membership in the association is available, but it is open to medical students and residents only.

American Medical Writers Association

40 West Gude Drive, Suite 101
Rockville, MD 20850-1192
301-294-5303
amwa@amwa.org
http://www.amwa.org

Visit this association's Web site to find links to useful conferences, products, and textbooks for medical writers. Students attending college can apply for student membership to gain benefits such as access to job postings and the ability to seek work via the association's freelance directory.

American Nurses Association

8515 Georgia Avenue, Suite 400
Silver Spring, MD 20910-3492
800-274-4ANA
http://www.nursingworld.org

This organization provides information on careers, an online journal about issues in nursing, a publications catalog, and links to state nursing associations.

American Organization of Nurse Executives (AONE)
Liberty Place
325 Seventh Street, NW
Washington, DC 20004-2818
202-626-2240
aone@aha.org
http://www.aone.org

Contact AONE for information on careers and continuing education.

American Physical Therapy Association (APTA)
1111 North Fairfax Street
Alexandria, VA 22314-1488
800-999-2782
http://www.apta.org

The APTA offers fellowships, awards, and scholarships to students enrolled in accredited physical therapy programs, as well as student membership for physical therapy students. Students who are still researching careers in physical therapy should visit the Association's "A Career in Physical Therapy" page under the Education section. The Web site also has a complete directory of accredited schools in the United States.

American Psychiatric Association
1000 Wilson Boulevard, Suite 1825
Arlington, VA 22209-3901
703-907-7300
apa@psych.org
http://www.psych.org

Visit the association's Web site for information on careers in psychiatry.

American Psychiatric Nurses Association
1555 Wilson Boulevard, Suite 602
Arlington, VA 22209-2405
866-243-2443
inform@apna.org
http://www.apna.org

Visit the association's Web site for answers to frequently asked questions about careers in psychiatric nursing, a list of graduate programs in psychiatric nursing, and information on membership for nursing students and scholarships.

American Registry of Diagnostic Medical Sonographers
51 Monroe Street, Plaza East One
Rockville, MD 20850-2400
301-738-8401
http://www.ardms.org

This Web site serves as a registration center for diagnostic medical sonographers planning to take certification exams. Practice exams, salary surveys, and a job board are also available.

American Society of Anesthesiologists
520 North Northwest Highway
Park Ridge, IL 60068-2573
847-825-5586
mail@asahq.org
http://www.asahq.org

The society offers career and educational information at its Web site.

American Society of Clinical Oncology
1900 Duke Street, Suite 200
Alexandria, VA 22314-3498
703-299-0150
asco@asco.org
http://www.asco.org

Visit the society's Web site for information on careers, a list of educational programs, useful publications, and job listings.

American Society of Human Genetics
9650 Rockville Pike
Bethesda, MD 20814-3998
866-486-4363
society@ashg.org
http://www.ashg.org

For various resources for high school, undergraduate, and graduate students, visit the society's Web site. The Careers in Genetics section provides undecided students with a description of jobs in the field. Also available is a training programs guide and resources for teachers at the K–12 level.

American Society of PeriAnesthesia Nurses
10 Melrose Avenue, Suite 110
Cherry Hill, NJ 08003-3696
877-737-9696
aspan@aspan.org
http://www.aspan.org

The society offers information on nurse anesthetist careers, scholarships for undergraduate and graduate nursing students, membership options, and information on continuing education.

Association for Gerontology in Higher Education (AGHE)
1030 15th Street, NW, Suite 240
Washington, DC 20005-1527
202-289-9806
http://www.aghe.org

Visit the AGHE's Web site to read *Careers in Aging: Consider the Possibilities,* which discusses the field of gerontology, careers available, how to select a program, and how to find jobs in aging. Also available online is scholarship information, special resources for students, and a searchable database of more than 750 gerontology programs.

Association for the Advancement of Medical Instrumentation
1110 North Glebe Road, Suite 220
Arlington, VA 22201-4795
703-525-4890
http://www.aami.org

The association offers information on certification and certification exam schedules, courses and seminars, and a searchable job board. Students in undergraduate or graduate programs can apply for student membership.

Association of American Medical Colleges
2450 N Street, NW
Washington, DC 20037-1126
202-828-0400
http://www.aamc.org

For a list of accredited U.S. and Canadian medical schools, career-related publications, and online resources for medical students, visit the association's Web site.

Medical students searching for a specialty will especially benefit from visiting the Careers in Medicine section.

Association of periOperative Registered Nurses
2170 South Parker Road, Suite 300
Denver, CO 80231-5711
800-755-2676
custserv@aorn.org
http://www.aorn.org

Visit the association's Web site to read *What is Perioperative Nursing?*, which details career options in the field. Its Web site also includes information on scholarships and grants, a perioperative nursing program online directory, and a list of questions to ask about perioperative nursing courses.

Association of University Programs in Health Administration
2000 North 14th Street, Suite 780
Arlington, VA 22201-2543
703-894-0940
aupha@aupha.org
http://www.aupha.org

Information on health care administration careers, scholarships for graduate students, and a database of educational programs is available on the association's Web site. High school students should visit the Prospective Student Info page, while college students will want to check out the undergraduate workshop and the internship postings.

Association of Women Surgeons
5204 Fairmount Avenue, Suite 208

Downers Grove, IL 60515-5058
630-655-0392
info@womensurgeons.org
http://www.womensurgeons.org

Visit the association's Web site for information on specialty options for women interested in surgical careers, student (medical) membership, and other useful resources.

Association of Women's Health, Obstetric and Neonatal Nurses
2000 L Street, NW, Suite 740
Washington, DC 20036-4912
800-673-8499
http://www.awhonn.org

This organization represents nurses who specialize in the care of women and newborns. Its members include neonatal nurses, OB/GYN and labor and delivery nurses, women's health nurses, nurse scientists, nurse executives and managers, childbirth educators, and nurse practitioners. It offers membership to nursing students and associate membership status for non-nurses who are "involved or interested in women's health, obstetric, or neonatal specialty."

Commission on Accreditation of Allied Health Education Programs
1361 Park Street
Clearwater, FL 33756-6039
727-210-2350
caahep@caahep.org
http://www.caahep.org

This organization accredits allied health educational programs. At the commission's Web site, searchable databases provide information about accredited programs available in each discipline as well as accreditations that are necessary.

Commission on Graduates of Foreign Nursing Schools (CGFNS)
3600 Market Street, Suite 400
Philadelphia, PA 19104-2651
215-222-8454
http://www.cgfns.org

The CGFNS offers support to foreign nurses who are interested in coming to the United States to work. Its Web site offers tips on finding a job, relocating to the United States, and selecting a recruiter. The organization also offers hospital location guides for a nominal fee.

Emergency Nurses Association (ENA)
915 Lee Street
Des Plaines, IL 60016-6569
800-900-9659
enainfo@ena.org
http://www.ena.org

Contact the ENA for information on careers, certification, and scholarships.

Medical Equipment and Technology Association Board
contact@mymeta.org
http://www.mymeta.org

The board offers membership for college students, as well as links to useful national, regional, and state biomedical science organizations at its Web site.

Midwives Alliance of North America
375 Rockbridge Road, Suite 172-313
Lilburn, GA 30047-5870
888-923-6262
info@mana.org
http://www.mana.org

Contact the alliance for information on the career of nurse midwife.

National Association for Practical Nurse Education and Service
PO Box 25647
Alexandria, VA 22313-5647
703-933-1003
jbova@napnes.org
http://www.napnes.org

This organization offers a certification program, information on continuing education, a professional journal, job listings, and membership to nursing students. It also hosts an annual convention.

National Association of Clinical Nurse Specialists
2090 Linglestown Road, Suite 107
Harrisburg, PA 17110-9428
717-234-6799
http://www.nacns.org

Contact the association for information on clinical nurse specialists careers, education programs, and membership for nursing students.

National Association of Health Care Assistants
2709 West 13th Street
Joplin, MO 64801-3647

417-623-6049
http://www.nagna.org

Visit the association's Web site for information on certification and employment opportunities and to participate in an online discussion forum.

National Association of Hispanic Nurses (NAHN)

1501 16th Street, NW
Washington, DC 20036-1401
202-387-2477
info@thehispanicnurses.org
http://www.thehispanicnurses.org

Contact NAHN for education and career information of particular interest to Hispanic nursing students, including scholarships, financial aid, and student services.

National Association of Neonatal Nurses

4700 West Lake Avenue
Glenview, IL 60025-1485
800-451-3795
info@nann.org
http://www.nann.org

The association provides information about neonatal nursing careers, employment, membership for nursing students, and publications at its Web site.

National Association of Nurse Practitioners in Women's Health

505 C Street, NE
Washington, DC 20002-5809
202-543-9693
info@npwh.org
http://www.npwh.org

Contact this organization to learn more about opportunities for nurse practitioners who specialize in women's health.

National Association of Pediatric Nurse Practitioners (NAPNAP)

20 Brace Road, Suite 200
Cherry Hill, NJ 08034-2634
856-857-9700
info@napnap.org
http://www.napnap.org

The NAPNAP's Web site provides information on the career of pediatric nurse practitioner and a list of educational programs.

National Association of School Nurses

8484 Georgia Avenue
Silver Spring, MD 20910-5604
866-627-6767
nasn@nasn.org
http://www.nasn.org

Visit the association's Web site for information on school nurse careers, certification, and membership for nursing students.

National Association of Science Writers Inc. (NASW)

PO Box 890
Hedgesville, WV 25427-0890
304-754-5077
info@nasw.org
http://www.nasw.org

Beginning science writers can find advice and job opportunities by visiting this association's Web site. Graduate students can apply to participate in the mentoring program, and writers under 30 can compete in a scholarship award competition. Student memberships are available to qualified college students.

National Black Nurses Association (NBNA)

8630 Fenton Street, Suite 330
Silver Spring, MD 20910-3803
800-575-6298
NBNA@erols.com
http://www.nbna.org

Contact the NBNA for education and career information of particular interest to African-American nursing students. The organization also offers information on membership for nursing students, scholarships, and job listings at its Web site.

National Conference of Gerontological Nurse Practitioners

7794 Grow Drive
Pensacola, FL 32514-7072
301-654-3776
admin@ncgnp.org
http://www.ncgnp.org

Visit the conference's Web site for a list of gerontological nurse practitioner educational programs.

National Council of State Boards of Nursing

111 East Wacker Drive, Suite 2900
Chicago, IL 60601-4277
312-525-3600
info@ncsbn.org
http://www.ncsbn.org

Contact the council for information on licensing and a list of state boards of nursing.

National Federation of Licensed Practical Nurses (NFLPN)

605 Poole Drive
Garner, NC 27529-5203
919-779-0046
http://www.nflpn.org

The NFLPN offers a national certification program, publications (including a professional journal), membership for nursing students and supporters of the federation, job listings, an online forum, and a list of state practical nursing associations.

National Gerontological Nursing Association

7794 Grow Drive
Pensacola, FL 32514-7072
850-473-1174
ngna@puetzamc.com
http://www.ngna.org

Contact this organization for information on gerontological nursing and certification.

National Health Council

1730 M Street, NW, Suite 500
Washington, DC 20036-4505
202-785-3910
info@nhcouncil.org
http://www.nationalhealthcouncil.org

The council offers *300 Ways to Put Your Talent to Work in the Health Field* ($18), which lists job descriptions and education requirements for health professions ranging from art therapists and clinical chemists to nurse practitioners and physicians. It also lists sources of information on training schools and financial aid programs for health professions.

National League for Nursing (NLN)
61 Broadway, 33rd Floor
New York, NY 10006-2701
212-363-5555
generalinfo@nln.org
http://www.nln.org

The league's goal is to "advance quality nursing education that prepares the nursing workforce to meet the needs of diverse populations in an ever-changing health care environment." Visit the NLN's Web site for career guidance materials (such as *A Career as a Nurse Educator*), information on approved schools of nursing, and links to other nursing organizations.

National League for Nursing Accrediting Commission Inc.
61 Broadway, 33rd Floor
New York, NY 10006-2701
212-363-5555
nlnac@nlnac.org
http://www.nlnac.org/Forms/
    directory_search.htm

The commission accredits all levels of nursing educational programs in the United States (including Puerto Rico), Guam, Scotland, and the Virgin Islands. Visit its Web site for a searchable database of these programs.

National Network of Career Nursing Assistants
3577 Easton Road

Norton, OH 44203-5661
330-825-9342
cnajeni@aol.com
http://www.cna-network.org

At its Web site, this organization offers a discussion board and information on state agencies that offer nurse-aide training programs.

National Organization for Associate Degree Nursing (NOADN)
7794 Grow Drive
Pensacola, FL 32514-7072
850-484-6948
noadn@puetzamc.com
http://www.noadn.org

Contact the NOADN for information on associate degree nursing programs.

National Society of Genetic Counselors
401 North Michigan Avenue
Chicago, IL 60611-4255
312-321-6834
nsgc@nsgc.org
http://www.nsgc.org

The society's Web site contains comprehensive information on genetic counseling in its Career section. Graduate students are eligible for student membership, and membership benefits include access to the job database and several professional publications.

National Student Nurses' Association (NSNA)
45 Main Street, Suite 606
Brooklyn, NY 11201-1099
718-210-0705

nsna@nsna.org
http://www.nsna.org

The NSNA's goal is to "organize, represent, and mentor students preparing for initial licensure as registered nurses, as well as those enrolled in baccalaureate completion programs." Its Web site provides information on nursing careers, surviving nursing school, scholarships, and resume writing and job hunting.

Oncology Nursing Society (ONS)

125 Enterprise Drive
Pittsburgh, PA 15275-1214
866-257-4ONS
customer.service@ons.org
http://www.ons.org

Contact the ONS for information on oncology nursing and certification. The society also offers scholarships to undergraduate and graduate oncology nursing students.

Society for Healthcare Consumer Advocacy

One North Franklin, Suite 31N
Chicago, IL 60606-3421
312-422-3851
shca@aha.org
http://www.shca-aha.org

For general information on health advocacy careers, visit the society's Web site.

Society of Diagnostic Medical Sonography

2745 Dallas Parkway, Suite 350
Plano, TX 75093-8730
800-229-9506
http://www.sdms.org

High school students who are thinking about a career in sonography will find this Web site's Career section especially valuable. It contains a complete overview of the profession, accredited programs database, an occupational outlook, and a career discussion forum. Student memberships are available for students who are enrolled in an accredited program, and scholarships are also available for those who are enrolled.

U.S. Department of Health and Human Services (USDHHS)

Bureau of Health Professions,
   Division of Nursing
5600 Fishers Lane, Room 9-35
Rockville, MD 20857-1750
301-443-5688
http://bhpr.hrsa.gov/nursing

Visit the USDHHS' Web site to find a variety of information on financial aid for those in the health professions, including scholarships and loans for disadvantaged students.

Index

Entries and page numbers in **bold** indicate major treatment of a topic.

A